Ace the OSCE

Ace the OSCE

First published in Great Britain in 2008 by

Ace Medicine Ltd

www.AceMedicine.com

British Library Cataloguing in Publication Data

A catalogue record for this book is available from the British Library

Library of Congress Cataloging-in-Publication Data

A catalog record for this book is available from the Library of Congress

Typeset by SNP Best-set Typesetter Ltd., Hong Kong

ISBN 978-0-9564647-0-5

Disclaimer

This book has been prepared mainly for use by medical students.

Although every effort has been made to ensure the accuracy of all material contained herein at the time of writing and filming, AceMedicine cannot guarantee the accuracy of all material at the time of publication. AceMedicine incurs no obligation to provide support or maintenance of updates to the material provided herein.

Whilst every effort is made to keep the material provided herein accurate and up-to-date, technical information changes rapidly and it is not possible to guarantee that all material is accurate at all times. If there is any doubt as to the accuracy of any material contained herein, the reader is responsible for verifying the accuracy using alternative information sources.

No part of this publication may be reproduced or transmitted in any form or by any means, or stored in any retrieval system of any nature without prior written permission, except for permitted fair dealing under the Copyright, Designs and Patents Act 1988, or in accordance with the terms of a license issued by the Copyright Licensing Agency in respect of photocopying and/or reprographic reproduction. Application for permission for other use of copyright material, including permission to reproduce extracts in other published works, shall be made to the publishers. Full acknowledgement of author and source must be given.

© AceMedicine 2007

Preface and how to use the book

In the run up to OSCE finals, everybody's greatest fear is not knowing what to expect in the exam.

"Will I pick up the signs?"

"What if I get the diagnosis wrong?"

This was our fear as final year medical students, so we brought together prize-winning teaching and examining clinicians to create an all-inclusive DVD and book pack.

The pack covers all the common OSCE cases that come up at finals and explains how to differentiate them.

The DVD shows you quickly and simply how to perform 37 examinations so you no longer have to read and try to understand from confusing books.

The book accompanies the DVD providing:

i.   Checklists

ii. Tips for diagnosis on inspection

iii. Causes and meanings of signs

iv. Detailed notes on abnormal findings and common differential diagnoses in colourful boxes

v.   How to link signs logically to come to a diagnosis

vi. Example examination case presentations

vii. Lists of investigations you'd ask for based on your clinical findings

Our pack will make you far more confident in the OSCEs as you will know exactly what to expect and won't be fazed by any OSCE patient.

How to use this pack

1. It would help to first watch an examination on the DVD then use the checklist to test yourself with.

2. Sit, read and memorize the detailed notes.

3. Watch the DVD again to be sure you understand each movement and manoeuvre.

4. It is best then to practice on a friend many times whilst timing yourself. Aim to complete each examination in 4–5 minutes.

5. Go out onto the ward and practice on real patients, actively looking for the signs you have read about.

6. Try and cover all the cases that we have listed as "Common OSCE cases" to be sure you have seen all the signs likely to be given to you at finals.

7. Practice presenting each case as is presented on the DVD to improve your skill and confidence.

8. Finally, walk into the exam with complete confidence as you will Ace the OSCE!

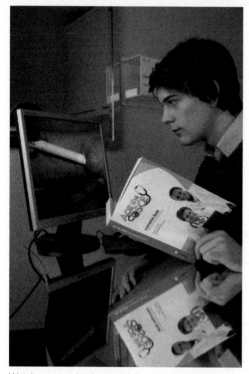

Watch an examination and follow it in the book

From all here at Ace Medicine: GOOD LUCK!

(If you'd like to publish with us, join the Ace Team or give us feed back please contact us via our website www.acemedicine.co.uk)

Acknowledgements

Editors:

Abtin Alvand MBBS, BSc (Hons), MRCS
Specialist Registrar in Trauma & Orthopaedic Surgery
Heatherwood & Wexham Park NHS Trust, Berkshire

Riaz Asaria BM MD FRCOphth
Consultant Ophthalmologist and Senior Lecturer
The Royal Free and University Hospital Medical School.

Ian Bickle B Bch, BAO
Specialist Registrar in Radiology
Sheffield Hospitals Trust

Warris A Bokhari MBBS, BSc (Hons)
Foundation year 1
Central Middlesex Hospital, London

Manish Chand MBBS, BSc (Hons), MRCS
Specialist Registrar in General Surgery
Wessex Deanery
& Neurosciences Tutor, Balliol College, Oxford University

Navtej Chahal MBBS, BSc (Hons), MRCP
Specialist Registrar in Cardiology, North West Thames Rotation
& Research Registrar, Northwick Park Hospital, Harrow.

Wayne Chicken MBChB, MRCS
Specialist Registrar in General Surgery
Northeast London Deanery

Tim Crook MBBS, BSc, PhD, MRCP
Specialist Registrar in Medical Oncology
Department of Medical Oncology, Charing Cross Hospital, London

Natalie Dabbas MBBS, BSc, MRCS
Specialist Training Registrar (ST2) in General Surgery
Wessex Deanery

Pooja Dassan MBBS, BSc (Hons), MRCP
Specialist Registrar in Neurology
London Deanery

Aruna Dias MBBS, BSc, MRCP
Specialist registrar in gastroenterology and teaching fellow at Newham University
& Hospital and clinical research fellow at Queen Mary School of Medicine and Dentistry,
University of London.

Preethi Gopinath MBBS, BSc, MRCS
Honorary Clinical Lecturer in Surgery
Queen Mary University of London
& Research Fellow, Institute of Cancer, London Deanery

Gerry J Gormley MD, MRCGP, DMH, DRCOG, PCertMedEd
Senior Clinical Academic in Clinical Skills
Clinical Skills Education Centre, Queen's University Belfast

Vanita Gossain BSc (Hons)
Final year medical Student
Royal Free & University College London Medical School

2 **Abhinav Gupta**
Medical Student
Royal Free & University College London Medical School

Maximillian Habibi BSc, MBBS, MRCP
Specialist Registrar in Infectious Diseases
Imperial College Healthcare NHS Trust

Fatima Z Jaffer BSc (Hons) MBBS
Foundation Year 1 Doctor
West Middlesex University Hospital, West London
North West Thames London Deanery

Emma Johnson MBBS, BA
Foundation year 1 Doctor
Central Middlesex Hospital, North West London Hospitals

Rajat Kapoor BMedSci (Hons), BM BS, DCH, MRCPCH
Specialty Registrar in Paediatrics and Child Health
London Deanery

Bhavesh Limbani MBBS, BSc
Foundation Year 1 Doctor
Whittington Hospital NHS Trust, London

Vishal Luther BSc (Hons)
Final year medical student
Royal Free & University College London Medical School

Gopal Metha BSc (Hons)
Medical Student
Royal Free & University College London Medical School

Michael Okorie BBS, MRCP (UK)
Specialist Registrar in Clinical Pharmacology & Therapeutics & General Internal Medicine
Centre for Clinical Pharmacology, UCL & UCL Hospitals NHS Trust

Derek Park MBChB, MRCS
Specialist Registrar in Trauma and Orthopaedics
NE Thames London Rotation

Aketa Patel BSc (Hons)
Final year medical student
Royal Free & University College London Medical School

Ameela Patel MBBS, BSc
Foundation Year 1 Doctor
University College Hospital, London

Zeudi Ramsey-Marcelle MBBS, MRCOG
Specialist Registrar in Obstetrics & Gynaecology
North London Deanery

Jeremy Rees
Consultant Neurologist
National Hospital for Neurology and Neurosurgery
Queen Square, London

Ben Rudge MBBS, MRCS
Specialist Registrar in Trauma and Orthopaedics
NE Thames London Rotation

Katherine Simpson BSc, MBChB, MRCP
Specialist Registrar in Diabetes & Endocrinology and General Internal Medicine
NW Thames London Deanery

Jennifer Townell MBBS
Foundation year 1
Whittington hospital
North central Thames

King Tin Tsang MBBS, BSc (Hons)
ST2 neurosurgery
London Deanery

Deirdre I. M. Wallace BSc Hons, RN, PGCE
Principal Clinical Skills Tutor UCL
UCL Medical School.

Tim Wickham MBBS, BSc, MRCP (UK), MRCPCH
Consultant Neonatologist
Barnet and Chase Farm Hospitals NHS Trust, London

Andrew Winter Diploma in Health Education RN/Child (APLS Provider)
Senior Staff Nurse in Paediatric Emergency Medicine
Chelsea and Westminster Healthcare NHS Trust, London

Special thanks:
Dr Dinesh Kapoor MBBS, DA, MRCGP
Senior Executive Partner
Leyton Healthcare medical Practice, Leyton

Caroline Paul
Clinical practice manager
Leyton Healthcare medical Practice, Leyton

Resuscitation Council (UK) 2007 Guidelines:
Adult Advanced Life Support
Adult Basic Life Support
Paediatric Basic Life Support

4 **7-Stage hand-washing technique**

Dedications

To my Mum and Dad who have supported and encouraged me whole heartedly through this production and have steered me through every obstacle with their wisdom and experience.

To my Brother, Sister and Sandeep for being so patient with me and for giving me your time, advice, unconditional love and support.

To Dr Dinesh Kapoor, Dr Eric Beck, Caroline, Vishaal, Hakeem, Sam H., Sam B., Tim C., Tim B., Aketa, Gopal and Abhinav. Thank you all for your huge efforts in creating this product and making it as useful as possible for students – this project would never have been possible without you.

Finally, thank you to Professor Irving Taylor, Professor John Rees, Deirdre Wallace, Sally Richardson, Dr Wayne Chicken, Dr Abtin Alvand, and every doctor who performed on the DVD or who contributed to the book. You have been a great team to work with and I look forward to working with you all again in the future.

Vanita Gossain

(Ace medicine producer)

Foreword

Many students find clinical examinations stressful and indeed the OSCE is often one of the most important parts of the overall assessment of clinical students. This book should help to allay those fears. It is extremely well written and appropriately focussed by a panel of genuinely enthusiastic teachers. It is a most professional work, which is highly relevant and its style is easily absorbable.

The DVD presentations are skilfully and professionally produced with experienced clinicians demonstrating with, importantly, real patients. The commentary is pitched at exactly the correct standard for finals.

Good luck in your exams!

Dr J Paul Dilworth MA DM FRCP
Sub Dean Student Welfare
Royal Free and University College Medical School
Consultant Physician

Contents list

Section 3: Specialities

Orthopaedics (Contributor: Abtin Alvand)

Obstetrics & Gynaecology

Paediatrics

Psychiatry

Dermatology

Radiology

Section 4: Practical Procedures
(Contributor: Sally Richardson)

Practical Skills

Life Support

House Officer Forms

How to revise for finals and how to present a case

Many final year medical students find the prospect of the OSCE a truly terrifying one and countless sleepless nights are spent in the preceding months agonising about the exam. The objective of the final OSCE is to assess your readiness and suitability to make the transition from medical student to doctor, with all the responsibilities that this entails. The OSCE examiners are looking for the evidence of this. They are not looking for the next professor of medicine or surgery. Despite this, many highly able candidates simply go to pieces during the exam and do not do themselves justice. So how can you minimise nerves on the day, remain calm in the febrile atmosphere leading up to the OSCE and arrive on the big day feeling relaxed yet focused? Whilst it is true that the examination room can be a pressurised and indeed intimidating environment, the key to avoiding these horrible feelings of dread is to ensure that you are adequately prepared. It really is as simple as that.

Preparation for any examination in medicine involves practice, practice and more practice of your clinical examination and presentational skills, combined with a good background knowledge of the subject. You must be completely familiar with clinical examination of the four big systems. Every doctor should be able to perform a competent and professional examination of the cardiovascular and respiratory systems, the abdomen and the peripheral and central nervous systems. It is absolutely essential that you practice your personal examination routine over and over again in front of your colleagues, friends and indeed anybody who will watch you. These may include fellow students, junior doctors on the firms you are attached to and, whenever you can persuade them, more senior clinicians. If you can't find anybody who matches this description, ask somebody else. You must be completely fluent and comfortable performing these examinations whilst being watched, and the only way to achieve such "autopilot" status is endless practice. It is always obvious when a candidate is not familiar with a particular examination, usually one they have performed only rarely as a student. For example, the majority of students can and do perform an acceptable clinical examination of the cardiovascular system, but many struggle with assessment of visual fields or a full cranial nerve examination, simply because they haven't (for some reason) done this very often on their clinical attachments and have not practiced it enough. So ensure that you really can examine, for example, the cranial nerves under pressure or assess the thyroid status of a patient while being critically observed. Practice, practice, practice. If you forget to do something in the exam, don't panic. You will not fail finals because you forgot to do vocal resonance when examining the chest, or omitted to check for peripheral oedema in the cardiovascular examination. You will, deservedly, fail if you don't show absolute respect for your patient and show a level of professionalism and maturity commensurate with your imminent progression to fully-fledged medical practitioner.

Another critical skill, frequently overlooked by medical students preparing for finals, is presentation of the cases you have examined. Again, as with examination skills, the key is endless practice until a fluent, concise presentation becomes second nature to you. Again, as with clinical examination, you must practice presenting to each other, to doctors and to anybody else who will listen. In each station, we have given examples of how typical cases might be presented. You will see that the presentation focuses on positive examination findings and how these might fit into a concise list of sensible differential diagnoses. Long lists of negative examination findings rarely impress the examiners. Our advice would be to include only the *relevant* negative findings in your presentation. If you have found no abnormalities on examination, then tell the examiners this, saying that your clinical examination was unremarkable. If there are signs that you have missed, the examiners may ask you to look again. This does not imply that you will fail the station, but gives you a second chance to find key signs that underpin your presentation and discussion of the case.

It is important when you have presented the case to the examiners to be able to offer a sensible differential diagnosis and to have some idea of how the case might be investigated. We have included lists of common OSCE cases, differential diagnoses of commonly appearing clinical signs and appropriate investigations for each station. Several important general points should be made about cases appearing in the OSCE and your presentation of the differential diagnosis and investigations.

1. Most of the cases appearing in finals will be patients who have chronic conditions with stable clinical signs. It is most unlikely that you will see an acutely unwell patient in the OSCE.

2. The majority of the cases will have common diagnoses. If a patient with good signs but a rare condition appears in the exam, you would not be expected to make the diagnosis but, rather, to present your findings in a sensible, rational manner and discuss investigation of the case.

3. If you are certain about a diagnosis, then it is acceptable to begin your presentation by stating this. For example, "This patient has aortic stenosis, as evidenced by the presence of a small volume, slow rising pulse and an ejection systolic murmur, loudest in held expiration, with radiation to the carotids". If you are not sure about the diagnosis, then simply present the positive examination findings and *relevant* negative ones and offer a sensible differential diagnosis. For example, "This patient has an ejection systolic murmur best heard in held expiration in the aortic area. The pulse volume is normal and there is no radiation of the murmur to the carotids. The heart sounds are normal, there are no stigmata of endocarditis, no sternotomy scars and no evidence of cardiac failure. The differential diagnosis includes aortic sclerosis, aortic stenosis and an aortic flow murmur".

4. Keep proposed investigations simple. For example, in cardiology the key investigations will almost always be an electrocardiogram (ECG), an echocardiogram and a chest X-ray together with simple blood tests such as full blood count to exclude anaemia and infection. Don't start your list of proposed investigations with complex, high technology techniques. Start simple and work up: just like it happens in real medicine.

Finally, we have compiled a list of ten simple tips to help keep you out of trouble on your big day.

Top ten OSCE tips

1. Smile on entering the room/cubicle and always maintain a pleasant, professional attitude throughout the OSCE. This creates a very favourable impression.

2. Speak clearly, concisely and confidently. Don't mumble your name/number.

3. We cannot overstate the importance of observation in each station. The silence may make you feel uncomfortable, but put on your wide-vision spectacles and look widely around the bed. The examiners will leave many clues for you, so take advantage of their generosity! In many cases, you can get a very good idea of the diagnosis simply by looking at and around the patient.

4. As we have emphasised above, the key to success in the OSCE is endless practice at examining patients and presenting the case.

5. You may not pick up every sign and you may not be able to formulate a unifying diagnosis. You will not fail because of this. Present your clinical findings in a professional manner when you have completed your examination, followed by a sensible differential diagnosis and simple, appropriate investigations.

6. If all else fails, go back to basics as this will help jog your memory.

   Examination: inspect, palpate, percuss, auscultate.

   Causes of: infection, inflammation, neoplastic, degenerative, autoimmune, metabolic, iatrogenic etc.

   Investigation. Start simple and work up. We have listed simple investigations for each station to help guide you.

7. For common cases, plan ahead how you would "manage" the patient. For example, pertinent questions you would ask in the history, signs to look for on other examination, investigation and treatment. Always try to include the buzzword "multi-disciplinary" in the management plans for your patients. This not only makes a favourable impression, but is exactly how modern medicine works in real life.

8. OSCEs are not, and never will be, a matter of life or death. Keep a sense of perspective about the exam and what is being assessed. Being nervous is natural but try and calm yourself down before you go in. You will not be faced with anything that you are totally unfamiliar with. And on the rare chance you are, it is certain that everyone will be as clueless as you are!

9. Ensure that you read the instructions carefully for each station and compose yourself before you begin. Remembering to adequately inspect the patient and the bedside environment should give you the time to compose yourself and go into "autopilot mode" as you start your examination.

10. It may sound ridiculous but try to enjoy the exam. It is your day, your chance to show the examiners (who are, after all, about to become your colleagues) that you are a safe, competent, pleasant and professional person who is ready to be given the title "Dr". The examiners are not looking for reasons to fail you. Far from it. The patients are volunteers and are happy to be there (unlike on the wards) and they often have fantastic signs, that you may have never seen an, indeed, may never see again. So enjoy the opportunity to exam these fantastic patients and to share your knowledge with the examiners. We wish you the very best of luck.

Section I
Medicine

Cardiovascular Examination

Summary

☐ Patient at 45 degrees, suitably exposed.

☐ Inspect for scars, chest asymmetry, malar flush and for congenital disorders.

☐ Inspect the hands for clubbing and stigmata of endocarditis.

☐ Examine the pulse and ask to measure the blood pressure.

☐ Inspect for corneal arcus, pallor, cyanosis and the high-arched palate of Marfan's syndrome.

☐ Assess the jugular vein pressure (JVP).

☐ Palpate the carotid pulse.

☐ Inspect the chest for scars and the cardiac apex.

☐ Palpate the apex and feel for heaves and thrills.

☐ Auscultate in the four areas of the precordium.

☐ Use appropriate manoeuvres for specific murmurs, e.g., held expiration for left-sided murmurs.

☐ Check for carotid bruit and carotid radiation of the ejection systolic murmur of aortic stenosis.

☐ Listen at the lung bases for bibasal crackles of cardiac failure.

☐ Finish off by feeling for peripheral oedema, pulsatile hepatomegaly, abdominal aortic aneurysm and the peripheral pulses.

Examiner's instruction

"Examine this patient's cardiovascular system and present your finding."

"Examine this patient's precordium and present your findings."

"This lady complains of increasing exertional shortness of breath and chest pain. Examine her cardiovascular system and try to establish the cause."

Common OSCE cases

- Atrial fibrillation
- Aortic regurgitation
- Prosthetic heart valve(s)
- Cardiac pacemaker
- Aortic stenosis
- Mitral regurgitation
- CABG

Key signs associated with common OSCE cases

- **Atrial fibrillation:** irregularly irregular pulse. Look for valvular pathology (particularly mitral valve) and hyperthyroidism. Yellow anti-coagulation book left at bedside.

- **Aortic stenosis:** small volume pulse, narrow pulse pressure, systolic murmur radiating to the neck, non-displaced apex.

- **Aortic regurgitation:** large volume, collapsing pulse, wide pulse pressure, early diastolic murmur, laterally displaced apex, visible neck pulsations.

- **Mitral regurgitation:** atrial fibrillation, pansystolic murmur radiating to the axilla.

- **Prosthetic heart valve(s):** sternotomy scar, systolic flow murmur, mechanical valve sounds (metal valves).

- **Coronary artery bypass graft (CABG):** midline sternotomy scar. The scar of saphenous vein harvest may be present.

- **Cardiac pacemaker/implantable cardiac defibrillator:** subclavicular scar with palpable mass below it.

Wh Wash hands

I Introduce yourself and identify patient

S Summarise what you would like to examine

P Permission

E Expose the chest

R Reposition – recline to 45-degree angle

S State of patient – well/unwell, old/ young, oxygen mask/ nasal cannula (What oxygen flow rate? Look at the flow meter on the wall.)

Signs around bed: nicotine replacement therapy, GTN spray, cardiac monitors, warfarin (anticoagulation) book.

General inspection

Stand at the end of the bed and look at the patient

- Scars – sternotomy, pacemaker, saphenous vein harvest
- Legs – scars and oedema.

Special signs

- Cyanosis/malar flush
- Body habitus – e.g., very thin patient potentially from hyperthyroidism with atrial fibrillation (AF) or Marfan's syndrome
- Tattoos/needle tracks – infective endocarditis
- Audible click – prosthetic heart valve
- Bruising – is the patient on warfarin for prosthetic heart valves or AF.

Diagnosis on inspection
Down's syndrome – congenital heart disease
Turner's syndrome – coarctation of the aorta
Marfan's syndrome – aortic regurgitation
Ankylosing spondylitis – aortic regurgitation

Hands

Inspect

"Can I have a look at your hands, please?"

- Clubbing

ACE TIPS
Ask the patient if they are in any pain before you touch them

Differential diagnosis: cardiology clubbing
Congenital cyanotic heart disease; atrial myxoma; infective endocarditis

- Stigmata of infective endocarditis – splinter haemorrhages, Osler's nodes, Janeway lesions
- Palmar erythema – hyperthyroidism, pregnancy, polycythaemia
- Tar staining
- Peripheral cyanosis.

Differential diagnosis: irregularly irregular pulse
Atrial fibrillation; ectopic beats; sinus arrhythmia (young patient)

Palpate

- Warmth – use the dorsal part of your hands
- Capillary refill – press pulp of finger for 5 seconds and count how long until the colour returns to a healthy pink (normal is <2 seconds)

- Radioradial delay – aortic coarctation
- Radial pulse – rate, rhythm, volume
- Collapsing pulse – a sign of AR:
  - Place the four fingers of the right hand across the palmar aspect of the distal forearm/wrist and lift the patients arm
  - In AR the pulse feels "tapping" on your fingers
- Indicate that you would like to take blood pressure:
  - If narrow pulse pressure – possible AS
  - If wide pulse pressure – possible AR.

> **Causes of atrial fibrillation**
>
> - Lone AF
> - Ischaemic heart disease
> - Hypertension
> - Mitral valve pathology
> - Hyperthyroidism (always offer to request thyroid function tests if your patient is in AF)
> - Alcohol
> - Sepsis (e.g., pneumonia)

Eyes

Inspect

"Look up" (you are looking for conjunctival pallor).

- Jaundice
- Corneal arcus, xanthelasma – hypercholesterolaemia/ senile arcus
- Pallor under eyelid – anaemia due to infectious endocarditis/ chronic disease, which may exacerbate underlying heart conditions.

Mouth

Inspect

- Central cyanosis under tongue – congenital heart disease
- State of dentition – infective endocarditis.

Neck

Inspect

- JVP – height and waveform
- If raised look carefully for ankle swelling and basal crackles at the end.

Palpate

- Carotid pulse – character and volume.

> **Differentiate venous from arterial pulsation in the neck**
>
> Venous pulsation:
>
> - Inspection – double pulse; changes with respiration
> - Palpation – non-palpable; disappears by finger pressure; hepatojugular reflex

---

> **Diagnosis from jugular vein pressure**
>
> • **Elevated** – congestive cardiac failure. Look for peripheral oedema, basal lung crackles
>
> • **Giant V wave** – coincident with the carotid pulse, is seen in TR
>
> • **JVP rises on inspiration** – constrictive pericarditis (Kussmaul's sign)

Chest

Inspect

• Scars:
- Midline sternotomy (CABG, aortic or mitral valve replacement)
- Left lateral thoracotomy (mitral valve replacement, valvotomy)
- Subclavicular (pacemaker or implanted defibrillator)

> **Diagnosis of midline sternotomy scar**
>
> Differentiate cardiac artery bypass graft (CABG) or a valve replacement:
>
> • **CABG** – look at the legs. Long, linear scars from saphenous vein harvest may be present, but in many patients vein harvest is from other sites (e.g., internal mammary artery) and legs scars are not present
>
> • **Prosthetic valve** – listen for prosthetic metal valve sounds

• Apex – visible, e.g., aortic regurgitation, thyrotoxicosis

• Pacemakers.

Palpate

• Apex beat – normally fifth intercostal space in the midclavicular line

• Heaves – left and right ventricular hypertrophy

• Thrills – palpable murmurs indicate severe valvular pathology
- If at the apex, think mitral regurgitation
- If in the aortic are, think aortic stenosis.

> **ACE TIP**
>
> If you see a midline sternotomy scar, you must listen very carefully for the characteristic sounds of a metal valve prosthesis, and identify which sound is abnormal. Don't overlook the possibility that the patient has a bioprosthetic valve replacement, which may be difficult to distinguish from normal heart sounds.

Heart sounds

S1: Closure of the mitral valve at the start of systole.

S2: Closure of the aortic (A) and pulmonary (P) valves at the start of diastole. S2 therefore has an aortic and a pulmonary component.

S3: Rapid ventricular filling in diastole as in heart failure and other hyperdynamic states.

S4: Atrial contraction attempting to fill a stiff, hypertrophic left ventricle as in severe aortic stenosis, hypertension and hypertrophic cardiomyopathy.

Diagnosis of displaced or heaving apex

• If laterally displaced, this is volume overload, seen in mitral and aortic regurgitation

• If not displaced but heaving, this is pressure overload (aortic stenosis)

Auscultate

Listen over the praecordium including the mitral, tricuspid, pulmonary, and aortic regions.

• Heart sounds I + II present/ prosthetic valve sounds

• Murmurs (diastolic/ systolic)

• Added sounds (e.g., S3, S4, opening snap, ejection click).

ACE TIP

It is essential to palpate the pulse when performing auscultation. The first heart sound coincides with closure of the mitral and tricuspid valves, which is when you will feel the pulse. Either the brachial or carotid pulse is acceptable, but ensure that the examiners can see that you are doing this.

Special manoeuvres

• Mitral stenosis:
  Roll patient to left lateral position
  Use bell of the stethoscope
  Listen in mitral area on expiration for mid diastolic murmur

• Mitral regurgitation:
  Roll patient to centre
  Use diaphragm of stethoscope
  Ask patient to hold breath in expiration
  Listen at apex for pansystolic murmur
  Listen for radiation to axilla

• Aortic regurgitation:
  Sit the patient up and lean them forward
  Using the diaphragm of stethoscope
  Listen at the left sternal edge on expiration for early diastolic murmur

- Aortic stenosis: Using the diaphragm of stethoscope

                       Listen in aortic area on expiration for a harsh ejection systolic murmur

                       Listen for radiation to the carotids

- Carotids: Using the bell of the stethoscope

                       Ask patient to briefly hold their breath

                       Listen for a carotid bruit

                       Listen for carotid radiation – murmur of aortic stenosis

- Lung bases: Listen for the crackles of pulmonary oedema.

Causes of ejection systolic murmur

- Aortic stenosis (small volume pulse, carotid radiation)

- Aortic sclerosis (normal volume pulse, no radiation)

- Hypertrophic cardiomyopathy (jerky pulse, double impulse at apex)

- Flow murmur

Tips on murmurs

- Left sided murmurs (aortic and mitral) are best heard in expiration

- Right sided murmurs (pulmonary and tricuspid) are best heard in inspiration

---

- Examine for sacral and ankle oedema
- Feel for peripheral pulses
- Examine for abdominal aortic aneurysm.

Finishing off

- Thank the patient
- Make sure patient is comfortable and offer to help cover them up
- Wash hands
- Present and consider age of patient in forming differential
- Summarise.

ACE TIP

It is unlikely that you will be confronted with a difficult murmur in the OSCE. The most probable murmurs (by far) are those of aortic stenosis and mitral incompetence. If you hear a murmur or the heart sounds of a prosthetic valve, look for and be seen to look for the stigmata of infective endocarditis.

Mention you would:

- Check for pulsatile hepatomegaly (tricuspid regurgitation) or tender hepatomegaly (congestive cardiac failure)

- Check for radio femoral delay
- Dipstick the urine
- Do a bedside BM (diabetes as a risk factor for cardiac disease)
- Perform fundoscopy (infective endocarditis, hypertensive/diabetic retinopathy)

Case presentation

"This patient has evidence of mitral regurgitation with a pansystolic murmur at the apex, which becomes louder on expiration and radiates to the axilla. He also has an irregularly irregular pulse, consistent with atrial fibrillation in keeping with the diagnosis of mitral valve disease. There is, however, no evidence of left ventricular failure or fluid overload."

"This patient has had surgery for a mitral valve prosthesis, as evidenced by the presence of a midline sternotomy scar and the absence of any scars in the legs. The first heart sound is prosthetic, consistent with closure of the mitral valve prosthesis. The valve is functional, and there are no stigmata of endocarditis or signs of cardiac failure."

Investigations

- Chest X-ray
- Electrocardiogram (ECG)
- Echocardiogram
- Cardiac catheterization
- Thyroid function tests in atrial fibrillation
- INR in atrial fibrillation and metal prosthetic heart valves.

⚙ Respiratory Examination

Summary

- ☐ Patient at 45 degrees, suitably exposed.

- ☐ Look for scars, chest asymmetry, deformity, tachypnoea, hoarse voice, cachexia, small stature, ptosis.

- ☐ Inspect the hands for clubbing, tar stains, cyanosis, and muscle wasting, CO_2 retention flap.

- ☐ Examine the pulse and the respiration rate.

- ☐ Inspect the eyes for pallor, and signs of Horner's syndrome.

- ☐ Look in the mouth for central cyanosis.

- ☐ Assess the jugular vein pressure (JVP).

- ☐ Palpate for the position of the trachea and for cervical lymphadenopathy.

- ☐ Inspect the chest for scars, asymmetry, deformity and radiotherapy tattoos and burns.

- ☐ Palpate the apex.

- ☐ Assess chest expansion.

- ☐ Percuss the chest, comparing the two sides.

- ☐ Auscultate the chest, comparing the two sides.

- ☐ Listen for vocal resonance.

- ☐ Repeat inspection, palpation, percussion, auscultation and vocal resonance on the back.

- ☐ To finish off, ask to see the observations chart, perform peak flow expiratory rate, measure oxygen saturations and look in the sputum pot.

Examiner's instruction

"This 64 years old lifelong smoker has become more breathless recently. Examine his respiratory system to establish the reason why."

"This 54 years old man is becoming progressively short of breath. Examine her respiratory system and find the cause."

"Examine this patient's respiratory system and present your findings."

Common OSCE cases

- Fibrotic lung disease
- Bronchiectasis
- Chronic obstructive airways disease
- Pneumonectomy/lobectomy

- Pleural effusion
- Cystic fibrosis
- Lung cancer
- Collapse

Signs associated with common OSCE cases

- **Fibrosing alveolitis:** clubbing, cyanosis, crackles.

- **Pleural effusion:** dull percussion note, reduced resonance, reduced breath sounds.

- **Cystic fibrosis (bronchiectasis):** young, small patient, clubbed, coarse crackles, purulent sputum

- **Obstructive airways disease:** hyper-inflated chest with reduced chest expansion, breathing with pursed lips, bounding CO_2 pulse, quiet breath sounds, wheeze, central cyanosis, tar-stained fingers, nebulizers and inhalers.

- **Lung cancer:** cachectic, clubbed, surgical scars, radiotherapy tattoos, pneumonectomy.

- **Pneumonectomy/lobectomy:** thoracotomy scar, decreased chest expansion, absent breath sounds. May be signs of lung cancer.

- **Collapse:** tracheal deviation, decreased chest expansion, dullness to percussion, quiet breath sounds.

Wh Wash hands

I Introduce yourself and identify patient

S Summarise what you would like to examine

P Permission

E Expose the chest

R Reposition – 45 degrees

S State of patient – well/unwell, old/young, rapid or laboured breathing, stridor, oxygen mask/nasal cannula (what oxygen flow rate?)

Signs around bed: inhalers/nebulisers/ peak flow meter/sputum pot (if there is one there, look in it).

Types of sputum

Black: smoking

Yellow/green: pneumonia/bronchiectasis

Red (haemoptysis): malignancy/ severe infection/ tuberculosis/ pulmonary embolism

Pink frothy: pulmonary oedema

Clues on inspection

Young: cystic fibrosis (bronchiectasis) with Hickman line/ Hickman line scar/ indwelling catheter indicating long-term antibiotic use.

Older: obstructive airways disease; lung cancer.

General inspection

Stand at the end of the bed and look at the patient

- Chest asymmetry (ask the patient to take a deep breath in)
- Weight loss, i.e., loose skin folds and protruding ribs (malignancy-associated cachexia)
- Neck, face and arm for swelling, plethora (superior vena-caval obstruction secondary to lung cancer)
- Eyes for ptosis (Pancoast tumour)
- Ask patient to cough – note nature e.g., dry/productive
- Look for nasal flaring, pursing of lips, use of accessory muscles, cyanosis (COPD)
- Look at the chest for deformities – often difficult but ascertain if barrel chest or not (COPD)
- Radiotherapy tattoos
- Do not miss surgical scars. Pneumonectomy is a popular case. The presence of a thoracotomy scar should point you to this diagnosis.

ACE TIP

The importance of observation cannot be overstated. The examiners will leave all kinds of clues for you, e.g., inhalers, peak flow charts, oxygen cylinders. So take your time, cast your eyes around the bed and gratefully accept these generous free gifts.

Differentiate asthma from chronic obstructive pulmonary disease

COPD features:

- Age of onset >35 years
- Smoking >10 years
- Breathless between attacks
- Sputum production
- No diurnal PEFR variation
- No/limited reversibility

Types of breathing patterns

Pursed lips on expiration – COPD

Accessory muscle use on inspiration – COPD

Kussmaul breathing: the deep, laboured breathing with normal or increased frequency – acidosis.

Hands

Inspect

• Clubbing – an important sign which, if present, immediately narrows down your differential. The respiratory causes of clubbing are listed in the box, and the commonest seen in finals are pulmonary fibrosis and bronchiectasis. If you suspect pulmonary fibrosis (PF), start thinking a little about the cause, which might be seen – i.e., do they have rheumatoid hands (Caplan's syndrome)?

Differential diagnosis for respiratory clubbing

• Fibrotic lung disease, e.g.:

  • Cryptogenic fibrosing alveolitis

  • Secondary to connective tissue disease (e.g., rheumatoid arthritis, systemic lupus erythematosus)

  • Secondary to occupation (e.g., asbestosis, silicosis)

• Suppurative lung diseases – cystic fibrosis, bronchiectasis, lung abscess, empyema

• Neoplasia – bronchial carcinoma, mesothelioma

• Nicotine stains – COPD, lung cancer
• Peripheral cyanosis – think particularly of pulmonary fibrosis and bronchiectasis
• Signs of steroid use (thin skin, easy bruising) makes a diagnosis of fibrotic lung disease more likely as this condition is rarely treated with anything else; but do not forget mismanaged overuse of oral steroids in long-standing COPD/asthma
• Wasting of the dorsal interossei (Pancoast's tumour) – if you see this, look for a Horner's syndrome
• Medic-alert bracelet – if on long-term steroids for obstructive airways disease.

"And now could you hold your arms out straight, as if you were stopping traffic? And just keep them there."

- CO_2 retention flap (coarse)/salbutamol tremor (fine). Ideally hold for 30 seconds, but in reality under OSCE conditions you don't need to. A salbutamol tremor would be obvious immediately, though CO_2 retention flap may take a little longer.

Palpate

- Radial pulse
  - Rate (count for 15 seconds, multiply by 4 to calculate beats per minute)
  - Rhythm – regular or irregular
  - Volume – a bounding pulse occurs in CO_2 retention.
- This is a convenient point in your examination to count the respiratory rate. As with the pulse, count for 15 seconds and multiply by 4.

Respiration rate

The normal respiration rate is about 12–20 breaths per minute (3–5 breaths in 15 seconds)

Tachypnoea is greater than 24 breaths per minute (6 breaths in 15 seconds).

Eyes

Inspect

- "Look up" (you are looking for conjunctival pallor)
- Horner's syndrome.

Differential diagnosis for atrial fibrillation in the chest station

- Comorbidity
- Pneumonia
- Bronchial carcinoma
- Massive pulmonary embolus

Horner's syndrome (signs)

- Miosis (constricted pupil)
- Ptosis
- Enophthalmos (sunken eye)
- Loss of sweating on face (anhydrosis)

Horner's syndrome (causes)

- Apical lung carcinoma (Pancoast tumour)
- Syringomyelia
- Trauma

Mouth

Inspect

"Please open your month for me and place your tongue to the roof of your mouth."

• Central cyanosis under tongue.

Neck

Inspect

• Jugular vein pressure (JVP) – elevated in cor pulmonale (right-sided heart failure secondary to chronic lung disease) e.g., end-stage COPD, severe bronchiectasis or fibrosis. If seen, make a mental note to inspect ankles fully for swelling and offer abdominal examination to look specifically for hepatomegaly, at the end

> **ACE TIP**
>
> The jugular vein pressure is ordinarily assessed with the patient resting comfortably at angle of 45 degrees.

• Cervical lymphadenopathy – some clinicians prefer to do this when you sit the patient forward to examine the back of the chest.

Differential diagnosis for cervical lymphadenopathy

Infection:

• Tuberculosis

• Tonsillitis

• Infectious mononucleosis

• HIV

• Toxoplasmosis

• Cytomegalovirus

Neoplasia:

• Lymphoma

• Leukaemia

• Metastatic carcinoma

Inflammatory diseases:

• Rheumatoid arthritis

• Sarcoidosis

• Systemic lupus erythematosus

Chest

Inspect

- Scars e.g. thoracotomy/ lobectomy/ pnemonectomy – lift both arms up separately as lateral scars may be difficult to see
- Radiotherapy tattoos
- Asymmetry, at rest and during breathing – i.e., if lung has been removed, this may be uneven
- Deformity

> **ACE TIP**
>
> Patients with previous pneumonectomy/ lobectomy are becoming more common in the exam.

> **Common chest deformity and causes**
>
> - Barrel chest – COPD
>
> - Pectus excavatum (sunken chest) – Marfan's syndrome
>
> - Pectus carinatum (pigeon chest) – rickets, chronic and severe childhood lung disease

Palpate

- Tracheal position – central or deviated. After feeling centrally, feel the grooves either side of the trachea and decide if they are equal. A deviated trachea may suggest volume loss (e.g., pneumonectomy/ lobectomy) so remember to look even more closely at the chest for scars. It may also be due to other causes of lung collapse (e.g., tumour or unilateral fibrosis)
- Apex beat. In healthy individuals, this is palpable in the mid-clavicular line in the fifth intercostals space.

"Please take a deep breath in for me . . . and again."

- Chest expansion – looking for asymmetry.

Percuss

"I'm now going to tap across your chest."

Compare the two sides – right and left:

- Clavicle
- Infraclavicular
- Chest (below nipple line)
- Axilla – upper and lower

> **ACE TIP**
>
> Many clinicians prefer to use the diaphragm of the stethoscope.

Auscultate

Compare the two sides – right and left:

- Supraclavicular (bell)
- Infraclavicular (diaphragm)
- Chest – below nipple line (diaphragm)
- Axilla – upper and lower (diaphragm).

Assess:

- Loudness – quiet breath sounds throughout: COPD (with wheeze)
- Quality – vesicular or bronchial (see table)

	Vesicular	Bronchial
Sound description	Soft	Harsh
Loudest phase	Breathing in	Breathing out
Longest phase	Breathing in	Breathing out

- Added sounds – wheeze, rubs and crackles
- Wheeze – can be inspiratory or expiratory
- Crackles:
    - Where are they?
    - Are they fine or coarse?
    - Do they clear on coughing – if so they are from residual secretions.

Describing crackles

Timing – crackles always occur during inspiration:

- Early inspiratory crackles originate in the bronchioles – COPD
- Late inspiratory crackles originate in the alveoli – pneumonia/ lung fibrosis

Sound – coarse or fine crackles:

- Coarse crackles are a sign of airway pathology – pneumonia/ bronchiectasis
- Fine crackles – Fibrosis and Failure (cardiac)

Causes of wheeze

- Asthma
- Chronic obstructive airways disease
- Heart failure (cardiac asthma)
- Lung cancer

Causes of pulmonary fibrosis

Apical lung fibrosis:

Progressive massive fibrosis

Ankylosing spondylitis

Sarcoidosis

Tuberculosis

Extrinsic allergic alveolitis

Elsewhere the causes are:

* Dusts (e.g., asbestos)

* Connective tissue disease

* Drugs (amiodarone, methotrexate)

* "Cryptogenic" fibrosing alveolitis

"Please can you now repeat 99, each time I touch your chest with the stethoscope."
* Vocal resonance:
    * Listen using the diaphragm of your stethoscope
    * Is it normal, loud (consolidation) or reduced (pleural effusion).

Causes of pleural effusion

Transudate (<30 g/l protein)

* Congestive cardiac failure

* Hypoalbuminaemia – liver cirrhosis, nephrotic syndrome, malabsorption

Exudate (>30 g/l protein)

* Infection – pneumonia, tuberculosis

* Neoplasia – bronchial carcinoma, metastases, mesothelioma

* Inflammation – sarcoid, rheumatoid arthritis, systemic lupus erythematosus

Back
"Please can you now sit forward for me, I'm going to repeat everything on the back."
* Palpate head and neck lymph nodes if you have not done this already
* Submental, submandibular, pre- and post-auricular, occipital, cervical and supraclavicular.

Inspect

- Scars
- Asymmetry
- Deformity.

Palpate

- Chest expansion.

Percuss:

Compare the two sides:

- Upper – percuss medially in the upper part otherwise you will hear dull sounds as you percuss directly over the scapulae
- Middle – midway between upper and lower sites of percussion
- Lower – above lower ribs
- Axilla.

Auscultate

Listen and assess breath sounds and vocal resonance in the same sites as for percussion.

Signs of common respiratory conditions

	Trachea	Expansion	Percussion	Auscultation	Vocal resonance
Consolidation	Central	Reduced	Dull ·	Bronchial Breathing, Coarse crackles	Increased
Lobar collapse	Pull towards lesion	Reduced	Dull	Reduced air entry	Decreased
Pulmonary fibrosis	Pulled towards lesion	Reduced	Dull	Fine crackles	Increased
Pneumothorax	Pushed away if tension (medical emergency)	Reduced	Hyper-resonant	Reduced breath sounds	Decreased
Pleural effusion	Pushed away if large	Reduced	Stony dull	Reduced breath sounds	Decreased

Finishing off
- Thank the patient
- Make sure patient is comfortable and offer to help cover them up
- Wash hands
- Present and consider age of patient in forming differential
- Summarise.

Mention that you would like to:
- Examine sputum pot and send the contents for culture
- Peak expiratory flow rate
- Inspect observation chart looking at oxygen saturation and temperature
- Request a chest radiograph if indicated

Case presentation
"On examination of this patient's respiratory system, he/she was comfortable at rest and breathing oxygen via nasal prongs using an oxygen bottle. There were inhalers present at the bedside; her pulse was 60 beats per minute, irregularly irregular. Her respiratory rate was 20 breaths per minute. There was no fine tremor of the outstretched hands, no clubbing or peripheral cyanosis. There was no evidence of anaemia, central cyanosis or lymphadenopathy. The chest was barrel shaped; expansion was reduced bilaterally. Percussion was resonant throughout. On auscultation, there were quiet wheezes throughout the chest, bibasal (fine/coarse) crackles, which were reduced after coughing. These findings are consistent with a diagnosis of chronic obstructive pulmonary disease."

"On examination of this patient's respiratory system, he/she was comfortable at rest. There was no clubbing, tar staining or fine tremor of the outstretched hands. The pulse was 60 beats per minute, irregularly irregular. Respiratory rate was 16 breaths per minute. The chest was symmetrical with no deformities. However, I note a left thoracotomy scar and a tattoo anteriorly, consistent with previous lung surgery and radiotherapy. Chest expansion was reduced on the left side and percussion dull at the left apex and stony dull at the left base. Breath sounds were bronchial at the left apex and absent at the left base. These findings are consistent with a lung neoplasm at the left apex, treated by surgery and radiotherapy. There is an associated left-sided pleural effusion."

Investigations
Fibrotic lung disease
- Chest X-ray (reticulo-nodular shadowing)
- High resolution CT scan
- Blood tests (elevated ESR, autoimmune markers)
- Pulmonary function tests.

Pleural effusion
- Chest X-ray
- Bronchoscopy, if indicated from the chest film
- Diagnostic aspiration (transudate or exudate?)
- Cytology (looking for malignant cells; culture; glucose, protein and LDH).

Bronchiectasis

- Chest X-ray (looking for ring shadowing)
- Sputum culture
- High resolution CT
- Consider genetic testing in the younger patient (cystic fibrosis?).

Obstructive airways disease

- Chest X-ray (hyper-expanded)
- ABGs – hypercapnia and hypoxia
- Blood tests (elevated white cell count is consistent with infection but many patients are on steroids, which can also cause an apparent neutrophilia).

Lung cancer

- Chest X-ray (may show discrete mass, collapse/ consolidation, pleural effusion, hilar lymphadenopathy)
- Cytology of sputum and/or pleural effusion
- Bronchoscopy and biopsy (for central lesions); CT-guided percutaneous biopsy for peripheral lesions
- Staging CT scan of chest, abdomen and pelvis
- Lung function tests if surgical intervention is planned.

Abdomen Examination

Summary

☐ Patient lying flat, suitably exposed.

☐ Inspect for scars, jaundice and tattoos.

☐ Look at the hands for clubbing, other nail changes, Dupuytren's contracture, liver flap.

☐ Check the arms for arteriovenous (AV) fistulae and other evidence of renal dialysis.

☐ Examine the eyes for pallor, jaundice and xanthelasma.

☐ Look in the mouth for ulcers, tongue changes and pigmentation.

☐ Palpate for supraclavicular and cervical lymphadenopathy.

☐ Look for spider naevi, gynaecomastia and hair distribution on the trunk.

☐ Inspect the abdomen for scar, stomas, striae, asymmetry and distension.

☐ Palpate systematically in all nine quadrants of the abdomen. Light initially, then deep.

☐ Palpate for hepatomegaly and splenomegaly.

☐ Attempt to ballot the kidneys.

☐ Percuss the abdomen to map the dimensions of any organomegaly.

☐ Check for ascites.

☐ Feel for an abdominal aortic aneurysm.

☐ Finish off by palpating for other lymphadenopathy, checking the external hernial orifices and assessing the presence of peripheral oedema.

☐ Ask to see the observations chart, check the BM, examine the external genitalia, perform a rectal examination and dipstick the urine.

Examiner's instruction

"Examine this patient's abdominal system and present your findings."

"This 48 years old patient has noticed that her eyes have become yellow. Examine her abdomen to establish the cause."

"This 64 years old man has noticed that his abdomen has become swollen. Examine him to find out why."

Common OSCE cases

- Jaundice
- Organomegaly
- Enlarged kidneys
- Abdominal scars and stomas
- Ascites
- Chronic liver disease
- Renal transplant

Key signs of common OSCE cases

- **Jaundice:** yellow discolouration of skin and sclera (look for clues to aetiology, e.g., hepatomegaly, stigmata of chronic liver disease, associated splenomegaly).

- **Ascites:** distended abdomen with shifting dullness (look for clues to aetiology, e.g., hepatomegaly, stigmata of chronic liver disease, evidence of neoplasia, congestive cardiac failure with raised JVP, peripheral and pulmonary oedema).

- **Organomegaly:** palpable liver and/or spleen (look for clues to aetiology e.g., myeloproliferative or lymphoproliferative disorders, liver cirrhosis, malignancy or congestive cardiac failure).

- **Chronic liver disease**: multiple stigmata (see information box below).

- **Enlarged kidneys**: unilateral or bilateral palpable kidney(s) +/– transplanted kidney +/– hepatomegaly (if polycystic disease).

- **Renal transplant**: arteriovenous fistula, right iliac fossa surgical scar, palpable transplanted kidney, signs of chronic immunosuppression.

Some eponymous signs in the abdomen

- **Murphy's:** tenderness and guarding in the right upper quadrant on inspiration = cholecystitis.

- **Rovsing's:** palpation in the left iliac fossa elicits tenderness in the right iliac fossa = appendicitis.

- **Grey Turner's:** bruising appearance in the flanks = pancreatitis.

- **Cullen's:** bruising appearance in the umbilicus = pancreatitis.

- **Courvoisier's:** if the gall bladder is palpable, the cause of painless jaundice is unlikely to be gall stones.

Wh Wash hands

I Introduce yourself and identify patient

S Summarise what you would like to examine

P Permission

E Expose the patient's chest and abdomen, keeping their underwear on. It is acceptable to pull back the lower garments to reveal level of the iliac crests so that the hernial orifices can be seen

R Reposition – recline to flat, head supported by a pillow

S State of patient – well/unwell, old or young, state of nutrition

   Signs around bed – sick bowls, feeding tubes, stoma bags, drains, e.g., bile.

ACE TIP

If the patient is at a 45-degree angle when you enter, it is acceptable to leave them in this position until you examine the abdomen itself because, to accurately assess the JVP, the patient needs to be at this angle.

Clues on inspection

Young: inflammatory bowel disease

Old: malignancy

Ethnic origin: thalassaemia causing hepatosplenomegaly and jaundice is more common in Greeks/Cypriots

---

General inspection
Stand at the end of the bed and look at the patient

- Gross abdominal distension
- Obvious scars
- Jaundice
- Dressings where biopsies may have been taken, e.g., lymph nodes, liver
- Tattoos, needle track-marks (viral hepatitis)
- Excoriations (scratch marks)
- Signs of long-term steroid use (cushingoid) and chronic immunosuppression that frequently occur in renal allograft and inflammatory bowel disease patients
- Signs of autoimmune conditions – auto immune hepatitis
- Slate-grey pigmentation – haemochromatosis
- Shortness of breath – alpha-1 antitrypsin deficiency.

Definition of jaundice ("icterus")

A yellow discoloration of the skin, sclera and mucous membrane caused by increased levels of bilirubin in the blood. Typically, the concentration of bilirubin in the plasma must exceed 50 μM (three times the upper limit of the normal range) for the coloration to be easily seen.

Hands

Inspect

ACE TIP

Ask the patient if they are in any pain before you touch them

- Clubbing – once you see clubbing, look for the other stigmata of chronic liver disease (CLD). Another common cause is Crohn's disease so make a note to palpate the right iliac fossa thoroughly for a mass.

Differential diagnosis for GI clubbing:

Inflammatory bowel disease; chronic liver disease; malabsorption, e.g. coeliac disease; GI lymphoma.

- Signs of iron deficiency – koilonychia (spooning of the finger nails). This is difficult to spot and pallor is an more obvious indicator so look carefully at the conjunctiva.
- Signs of chronic liver disease:
  - Leuconychia -indicating hypoalbuminaemia
  - Palmar erythema – indicating hyper-dynamic circulation due to increased oestrogen circulation
  - Dupuytren's contracture.

Differential diagnosis for palmar erythema:

Chronic liver disease; thyrotoxicosis; pregnancy

Differential diagnosis for Dupuytren's contracture:

Chronic liver disease; congenital ulnar nerve palsy

"And now could you hold your hands like this, as if you were stopping traffic? And just spread your fingers and keep them there."

- Liver flap – this is a coarse tremor that may involve some but not necessarily all of the fingers. This indicates encephalopathy. You are very unlikely to get this in finals, but you will see it in your practicing career.
- Look for (and feel) in the arms, particularly in the antecubital fossa, for AV fistulae in renal replacement therapy patients.

Signs of chronic liver disease

- Clubbing
- Leuconychia
- Palmar erythema
- Dupuytren's contracture
- Telangiectasia
- Enlarged parotids
- Spider naevi
- Gynaecomastia
- Hepatomegaly
- Testicular atrophy
- Axillary hair loss

ACE TIP

As well as looking for Dupuytren's, when you ask the patient to turn over their hands for you, run your thumbs neatly across the palmer aspect to feel for fibrosis of the aponeurosis. This will stop you missing it and also show the examiners that you are thorough.

Definition of arteriovenous fistula

An AV is a surgically created connection between an artery and a vein in the forearm used for haemodialysis treatments. Its presence must alert you to the possibility of a transplanted kidney.

Face and neck

Inspect

Eyes

"Look up" (you are looking for conjunctival pallor). "Look down" (you are looking for jaundice).

- Jaundice (conjugated bilirubin often gives more intense skin pigmentation as a results of its water solubility)
- Pallor under eyelid – anaemia differential diagnosis: malignancy, Crohn's disease, celiac disease
- Xanthelasma – seen in primary biliary cirrhosis (most often middle-aged women with fantastic CLD signs).

Causes of anaemia

Microcytic ("FAST"):

- **F**e deficiency
- **A**naemia of chronic disease
- **S**ideroblastic anaemia
- **T**halassaemia

Normocytic:

- Anaemia of chronic disease
- Combined haematinic deficiency (iron and folic acid)
- Chronic renal failure
- Bone marrow failure

Macrocytic:

- Megaloblastic (B12, folate deficiency)
- Myelodysplasia
- Alcohol abuse
- Chronic liver disease
- Haemolysis (jaundice)
- Hypothyroidism
- Cytotoxic drugs

Causes of jaundice

Prehepatic:

- Haemolysis
- Gilbert's

Hepatic:

- Alcoholic liver disease
- Viral hepatitis
- Neoplasia
- Drugs:
  - Tuberculosis medication
  - Amiodarone
  - Amitriptyline
  - Nonsteroidal anti-inflammatories

Cholestatic:

- Gall stones in the common bile duct
- Carcinoma of the head of the pancreas
- Primary biliary cirrhosis
- Drugs:
  - Oral contraceptive pill
  - Phenothiazines
  - Macrolides
  - Penicillins
  - Nitrofurantoin
  - Gold

Mouth

- Glossitis – vitamin B deficiencies
- Angular stomatitis – anaemia
- Apthous ulcers – inflammatory bowel disease, coeliac disease

- Oral candidiasis – steroid therapy, immunosuppression
- Telangiectasia – hereditary haemorrhagic telangiectasia, red vascular marks most often seen in older patients
- Pigmentation (dark/black freckles) around the mouth – Peutz–Jeghers syndrome.
- Parotid enlargement – sign of excess alcohol use.

Neck

"Could you please sit forward whilst I feel for glands in your neck. Can you tilt your head slightly upwards and look straight ahead?"

- Examine for cervical lymphadenopathy. Feel for Virchow's node (Trousier's sign). This is the presence of localized lymphadenopathy in the left supraclavicular fossa and may be indicative of gastric carcinoma.

ACE TIP

While the patient is sitting forward, you can take the opportunity to quickly check for the presence of sacral oedema (chronic liver disease, congestive cardiac failure).

Differential diagnosis for cervical lymphadenopathy

Infection:

- Tuberculosis
- Tonsillitis
- Infectious mononucleosis
- HIV
- Toxoplasmosis
- Cytomegalovirus

Neoplasia:

- Lymphoma
- Leukaemia
- Metastatic carcinoma

Inflammatory diseases:

- Rheumatoid arthritis
- Sarcoidosis
- Systemic lupus erythematosus

Chest

Inspect

- Spider naevi – a sign of hyperoestrogenism in chronic liver disease. As a general rule they are found in the distribution of the IVC so look particularly on the left side (arms, chest, back). More than three is significant.
- Gynaecomastia – often tender.
- Hair distribution – another CLD sign due to the increased oestrogen (the damaged liver can not metabolise it adequately so the blood levels increase). Look for loss of hair in the axilla and groin.

Causes of gynaecomastia

- Cirrhosis
- Drugs (spironolactone, digoxin, cimetidine, cannabis)
- Klinefelter's syndrome
- Testicular cancer

Common abdominal scars

- Right upper quadrant – cholecystectomy
- Right iliac fossa – appendicectomy
- Midline – laparotomy
- Suprapubic – pelvic surgery
- Loin – renal surgery
- Midline laparotomy scar plus linear 3 inch scar in the left iliac fossa – possible bowel resection and reversal of colostomy

Abdomen

Inspect

* Scars

* Striae – long-term corticosteroid use and chronic liver disease

* Caput medusa, a sign of portal hypertension – venous flow can be seen going away from the umbilicus as the portal blood backs up due to the high pressure in the portal system

* Distension – clues to ascites being present is fullness in both flanks and everted umbilicus (this requires significant volume of ascites to be present). Look at the ankles now for oedema

* Stomas – not something that you will fail to see, but again you must mention it. 1) Gently lift the bag to discriminate between single or double lumen or flush/spouted; 2) Look at the bag contents

* Scratch marks – **s**een in PBC due to intractable pruritus (itch) resulting from deposition of bile salts in the skin

* Collateral blood vessels on the anterior abdominal and/or chest wall

* Asymmetry – masses/ organomegaly can sometimes be seen.

Stoma	Ileostomy	Colostomy
Location	Right lower quadrant	Left lower quadrant
Contents	Liquid	Semi-solid
Appearance	Spouted	Flat with the skin
Indication	Ulcerative colitis	Colorectal cancer, diverticulitis, volvulus

6 F's of distension

Fat

Faeces – constipation

Flatus – obstruction

Fluid – ascites

Fetus

Filthy big tumour

Causes of pruritus

* Jaundice (in the abdominal station, itch is frequently associated with primary biliary cirrhosis).

* Chronic renal failure

* Hodgkin's disease

* Dermatological disease (urticaria, eczema)

* Thyroid disease

* Polycythaemia

* Iron deficiency anaemia

Palpate

"I'm now going to feel your tummy, first gently then a little firmer – let me know if you get any pain. Are you in any pain now?"

- Kneel beside patient
- Warm your hands
- Look at the patient's face as you palpate and percuss

Systematic light palpation

Begin palpation at point furthest away from site of pain specified by patient

- Tenderness
- Guarding, rebound tenderness, rigidity – not commonly seen in OSCES!
- Gross masses

Deep palpation

- Localised masses – if you feel a mass, think about how you will describe it. As for any other lump you need site, size, shape, contour, consistency, tender, pulsatile, fluctuating, etc. For example: "There is a mass felt in the epigastric region that is approximately 10 cm in diameter with a rounded shape. It was hard, smooth, non-tender and non-fluctuating. It was not attached to the overlying skin and moved with respiration".

> **ACE TIP**
>
> Try to keep your hand in contact with the skin at all times so that your palpation is thorough. You should flex the fingers at the MCP joints and palpate in all 4 quadrants / 9 areas of the abdomen. The examiner will be checking to ensure that you palpate all over.

Abdominal masses

Right upper quadrant (RUQ)	Epigastrium	Left upper quadrant (LUQ)
Hepatomegaly	Stomach carcinoma	Splenomegaly
Gallbladder carcinoma	Pancreatic carcinoma/	Stomach carcinoma
Renal masses	pseudocyst	Pancreatic carcinoma/
Ascending colonic masses		pseudocyst
		Renal masses
		Descending colonic masses
	Umbilical	
	Abdominal aortic aneurysm	
	Transverse colonic masses	
Right lower quadrant (RLQ)	**Supra pubic**	**Left lower quadrant (LLQ)**
Appendix mass/abscess	Bladder retention	Renal masses
Renal masses	Bladder carcinoma	Ovarian cyst, malignancy
Ovarian cyst, malignancy	Uterine fibroids,	Ascending colonic masses
Ascending colonic masses	carcinoma	
	Pregnancy	

> ### ACE TIP
>
> Transplanted kidneys commonly appear in finals. There is usually a diagonal scar in the RIF, which is about three times the length of an appendicectomy scar and has a palpable kidney beneath it. If you feel a transplanted kidney and have not noticed AV fistula/ chronic ambulatory peritoneal dialysis scar sites/steroid side effects – look again. You must carefully examine these patients for the effects of chronic immunosuppression. For example, ciclosporin often causes gum hypertrophy and coarse tremor. Look also for evidence of long-term steroid use and skin cancers.

Special manoeuvres

"I'd now like you to take some deep breaths in for me, when I say so, as I feel your tummy."

Hepatomegaly

- Liver edge:

    Move progressively from right iliac fossa up to right costal margin. Wait on inspiration to feel a knock from the liver edge against the border of the index finger.

- Liver span:

    Percuss from right iliac fossa up towards right costal margin looking for transition of note from tympanic to dull – lower edge. Percuss from right upper chest down towards right iliac fossa looking for transition of note from resonant to dull – upper edge. This is important because the upper border of the liver starts at the fourth costal cartilage but may be displaced downwards in hyper-expanded lungs (e.g., COPD), which may fool you into thinking it is enlarged.

If you feel the liver, estimate the size and, when presenting, comment particularly on its smoothness, tenderness, pulsatility and movement on respiration.

> ### Differential diagnosis for hepatomegaly
>
> Common: carcinoma; cirrhosis; congestive cardiac failure
>
> Interesting (less common): infective (HBV, HCV, EBV, CMV); infiltrative (Wilson's disease, haemochromatosis); immunological (primary biliary cirrhosis)

Splenomegaly

- Move progressively from right iliac fossa up to the left costal margin. Wait on inspiration to feel a knock from the spleen against the tips of the fingers. Percuss from right iliac fossa up to left costal margin, ensuring to feel laterally also.

Differential diagnosis for splenomegaly

Massive: myelofibrosis; chronic myeloid leukaemia; malaria; leishmaniasis; Gaucher's disease

Moderate: lymphoproliferative disorders (lymphoma, CLL); amyloid; portal hypertension

Tip: haemolysis; infection (EBV, CMV, HBV endocarditis); sarcoidosis, rheumatoid arthritis

2

Differential diagnosis for hepatosplenomegaly

Myelo-/ lymphoproliferative disorders; haemolysis; infiltrative diseases (sarcoidosis, haemochromatosis); portal hypertension

Definitions

Myeloproliferative disorders: a group of diseases of the bone marrow in which there is abnormal proliferation of one of the cell lineages (myeloid, erythroid and megakaryocyte), including myelofibrosis, chronic myeloid leukaemia, primary polycythaemia, essential thrombocythaemia.

Lymphoproliferative disorders: disorders in which lymphocytes are produced in abnormal quantities, including lymphoma, leukaemia.

Enlarged kidney

- Right kidney – slide left hand under patient to renal angle, below 12th rib but above posterior iliac crest. Press down with right hand but do not feel too laterally as the kidneys are paravertebral. Flex the fingers of the left hand to feel an enlarged kidney knock the right hand (balloting).
- Left kidney – use the opposite hands to ballot the left kidney.

1

ACE TIP

Polycystic kidneys are common and can be confusing on palpation as they may be enormous and seem to fill the whole abdomen. They may feel lumpy and cystic also but some do not. There is often associated hepatomegaly (cysts also affect the liver). Look for the surgical scar of contra-lateral nephrectomy. You MUST ask to measure the blood pressure. Is there a transplanted kidney?

Differential diagnosis for enlarged kidneys

Unilateral: renal cyst; hydronephrosis; renal cancer

Bilateral: polycystic kidney disease; bilateral hydronephrosis; bilateral renal cancers

Differentiate the kidney from the spleen

	Spleen	Kidney
Upper border palpable	No	Yes
Notch	Yes	No
Ballotable	No	Yes
Movement on inspiration	Down + towards RIF	Down
Percussion note	Dull	Resonant

Ascites

Even if you do not suspect ascites/distension, always examine for shifting dullness):

* With your fingers in the coronal plane, percuss from umbilicus to distal flank looking for transition in note from tympanic to dull (suggesting fluid accumulation in the peritoneal cavity). If transition is evident, keep the percussed finger at this point and ask the patient to roll towards you. Hold this position for 10 seconds, allowing any fluid to "shift". Look for change in note from dull to tympanic on repercussion of the finger.

ACE TIP

With gross ascites, a fluid thrill can also be elicited. Ask the examiner to place their hand centrally, little finger down in midline. Place your right hand on the left side of the patient's abdomen and flick firmly with your left hand. A lot of fluid needs to be present for this sign to be positive.

Common causes of ascites

Cirrhosis; cancer (particularly pelvic malignancy); congestive cardiac failure

---

Classification of ascites

Transudate (<30 g/l protein) – congestive cardiac failure

Hypoalbuminaemia – cirrhosis, nephrotic syndrome

ACE TIP

The commonest causes of hepatomegaly are also the commonest causes of ascites. So one simple list covers two common exam cases (which frequently coexist of course).

Abdominal aortic aneurysm

- Place the fingers of both hands either side of the midpoint between the xiphisternum and umbilicus – fingers are pushed upwards and outwards (expansile).

Auscultation

Bowel sounds

- Present or absent
- Tinkling – obstruction (unlikely to be in finals)
- Bruits – renal, liver (if hepatomegaly) and over an abdominal aortic aneurysm (AAA) if felt. If you feel an AAA, offer to do a full peripheral vascular examination at the end.

Finishing off

- Thank the patient
- Make sure patient is comfortable and offer to help cover them up
- Wash hands
- Present and consider age of patient in forming differential
- Summarise.

Mention you'd like to do the following:

- External hernial orifices (if not already done)
- Rectal examination – palpating for masses, stool, feeling prostate, blood, etc.
- External genitalia – hernias may go into the scrotum
- Urine dipstick looking for evidence of infection, haematuria and proteinuria
- Other lymphadenopathy (if appropriate, i.e., other nodes/organs felt)
- Observation chart – temperature, blood pressure (kidney problems may cause or be due to hypertension)
- BM reading – liver/pancreatic disease can cause glucose disturbances.

Case presentation

"In summary, this gentleman is comfortable at rest. He presents with an obvious fistula in his left forearm and he has a scar in his right iliac fossa, consistent with a renal transplant. There is a non-tender mass in the right iliac fossa, consistent with a transplanted kidney. I could find no evidence of hepato- or splenomegaly, and there were no other signs of chronic liver disease. I think this gentleman has a transplanted kidney in the right iliac fossa. There are no stigmata of long-term corticosteroid use or chronic immunosuppression. There are no signs of chronic renal failure."

"In summary this lady has no obvious signs of peripheral stigmata of chronic liver disease. She has an obvious midline scar and one in the right iliac fossa with the presence of a stoma in the left iliac stoma. This is consistent with a colostomy because it is flush to the skin in the left lilac fossa, and it has formed bowel content coming through it. There was also the presence of an incisional hernia, which was demonstrated on examination."

Investigations

Jaundice

- FBC – looking for macrocytosis
- Reticulocyte count and Coombs' test to exclude haemolysis

- Ultrasound scan of abdomen (cause of obstructive jaundice?; fatty liver?; evidence of cirrhosis?)
- Liver function tests – cholestatic or hepatitic jaundice.
- INR
- Serology for HBV, HCV, EBV and CMV
- Antimitochondrial antibodies (PBC).

Ascites

- Diagnostic tap sent for:
  - Cytology: malignant cells
  - Biochemistry: protein >30 g/l: exudate
    - protein <30 g/l: transudate
  - Microbiology
- Ultrasound scan of abdomen: looking for evidence of liver and ovarian pathology

Hepatomegaly

- FBC
- Liver function tests
- INR
- Ultrasound scan of abdomen
- If malignancy suspected:
  - CT scan of chest, abdomen and pelvis
  - Colonoscopy, endoscopy
  - CT or ultrasound-guided biopsy
- If cardiac failure suspected
  - Echocardiogram
- If cirrhosis suspected:
  - Serology for HBV and HCV
  - Antimitochondrial antibodies (PBC)
  - Caeruloplasmin (Wilson's disease)
  - Ferritin +/– DNA sequencing of HFE gene
  - Alpha-1 antitrypsin.

Chronic liver disease

- Investigations as above for cirrhosis.

Enlarged kidneys/renal transplant

- Urea and electrolytes
- Ultrasound abdomen: looking for evidence of cysts/ malignancy/ hydronephrosis
  - Urine cytology
- Staging CT scan if renal malignancy is suspected.

Splenomegaly

- Ultrasound abdomen: to confirm splenomegaly
- FBC, bone marrow analysis (aspirate and trephine), serum LDH
- Staging CT scan.
- Tissue diagnosis: biopsy of pathological lymph node(s)
- Thick and thin blood films (malaria)
- Viral serology: EBV, CMV, HBV.

⊙ Neurology: Peripheral Nervous System Examination – Introduction

Examiner's instruction

"Examine the motor neurological system in the arms of this patient and present your findings."

"This young woman has had several episodes of weakness in her legs. Examine her legs and anything else relevant."

"This gentleman describes increasing difficulty in walking. Examine his lower limbs and find out why."

Common OSCE cases

- Multiple sclerosis
- Stroke
- Peripheral neuropathy
- Proximal myopathy
- Motor neuron disease
- Parkinson's disease (see separate station)
- Myaesthenia gravis
- Carpal tunnel syndrome
- Ulnar nerve palsy
- Radial nerve palsy

Key signs associated with common OSCE cases

- **Multiple sclerosis:** young, UMN spasticity in limbs, hyper-reflexic, cerebellar signs, internuclear ophthalmoplegia, optic atrophy

- **Stroke**: older, characteristic posture, hemiplegic, co-existent cranial nerve deficits

- **Peripheral neuropathy**: bilateral, symmetrical loss of sensation +/– motor weakness

- **Proximal myopathy:** weakness and wasting of proximal muscles with preservation of distal muscles

- **Motor neuron disease:** may have co-existent upper and lower motor neuron signs, fasciculations, no sensory signs, dysarthria, bulbar or pseudobulbar palsy

- **Myaesthenia gravis**: ptosis, diplopia, fatigueable weakness

- **Carpal tunnel syndrome**: compression of the median nerve, wasting of thenar eminence; weakness of thumb flexion, abduction and opposition; sensory loss over lateral three and a half fingers

- **Ulnar nerve palsy:** wasting of the small muscles of the hand. ulnar claw hand at fourth and fifth fingers

Investigations

- **Multiple sclerosis:** MRI brain, cerebrospinal fluid (CSF) analysis looking for oligoclonal bands, visual evoked potentials
- **Spastic paraparesis:** MRI brain (multiple sclerosis); MRI spine (cord compression)
- **Hemiplegia:** CT brain (stroke)
- **Peripheral neuropathy:** urine dipstick (glucose); serum B12 and folate; FBC (macrocytosis in chronic alcohol abuse); liver function tests including gamma-glutamyl transpeptidase (γGT); urea and electrolytes (chronic renal failure); CXR (malignancy)
- **Proximal myopathy:** investigations are guided by clinical suspicion of the likely underlying cause – urine dipstick (glucose in diabetic amyotrophy); thyroid function tests; ESR (inflammatory myopathies); CXR (lung cancer associated neuropathy); muscle biopsy may be required
- **Motor neuron disease:** a clinical diagnosis, but electromyography shows fasciculations
- **Pseudobulbar palsy:** MRI brain (to exclude multiple sclerosis); CT brain (to exclude stroke); electromyography (shows fasciculations in motor neuron disease)
- **Bulbar palsy:** electromyography (shows fasciculations in motor neuron disease)
- **Myaesthenia gravis:** edrophonium test; serum acetylcholine receptor antibodies
- **Carpal tunnel syndrome:** nerve conduction studies, then establish the cause. Investigations according to clinical suspicion – hCG (pregnancy); thyroid function tests; glucose tolerance test (acromegaly)
- **Ulnar nerve palsy:** nerve conduction studies
- **Radial nerve palsy:** nerve conduction studies.

Neurology: Motor Examination of the Arms

Summary

☐ Patient comfortable with arms and legs suitably exposed.

☐ Starting in the upper limb, inspect for wasting, fasciculation and tremor.

☐ Check for pronator drift and rebound phenomenon.

☐ Assess tone at the wrists and elbows.

☐ If there is increased tone, check for the presence of clonus

☐ Test power: shoulder abduction, elbow flexion, elbow extension, finger flexion, finer extension, abduction of the thumb.

☐ Check biceps, triceps and supinator reflexes.

☐ Assess coordination (dysdiadochokinesis and finger–nose test).

Wh Wash hands

I Introduce yourself and identify the patient

S Summarise what you are going to do

P Permission

E Exposure of patient. Expose the arms and trunk

R Reposition the patient

S State of patient – old/young, well/unwell, catheter, nasogastric tube, Signs around bed – walking stick, wheelchair.

ACE TIP

Hemiplegic patients have a characteristic posture, with the arm held at the side and the elbow, wrist and fingers flexed. The leg is extended at hip and knee and the foot plantar flexed. If you see this appearance, you know the diagnosis immediately (stroke).

General inspection

- Muscle wasting (generalised, proximal or single muscle)
- Fasciculations
- Posture
- Temor
- Face – dystrophia myotonica, parkinsonism, Horner's syndrome.

ACE TIP

Ask the patient if they are in any pain before you touch them

---

Start by looking for pronator drift (identifies an upper motor neurone condition)and rebound phenomenon (identifies cerebellar disorder).

ACE TIP

The presence of fasciculations is a strong pointer to the diagnosis of motor neuron disease.

Tone

- Assess tone by flexing and extending at the elbow joint, pronation and supination of the forearm and flexion and extension at the wrist.
- At this point, assess for clonus by rapidly pronating the forearm and note oscillations. More than three beats is abnormal and is an upper motor neuron (UMN) sign.

Power

Assess power in the following muscle groups:

- Deltoids – shoulder abduction: ask patient to stop you pushing down.
- Biceps – flexion at the elbow: ask patient to stop you pulling the arm.
- Triceps – ask the patient to flex the elbow and stop you pushing the arm.
- Extensor digitorum – ask the patient to extend fingers and stop you pushing them down.
- Flexor digitorum – ask the patient to make a fist and stop you opening it.
- Abductor pollicis brevis – ask the patient to point thumbs to the ceiling against your resistance.

Grade power using the MRC scale.

Root	Nerve	Muscle group tested	Muscle action tested
C5	Axillary	Deltoid	Shoulder abduction
C5, C6	Musculocutaneous	Biceps	Elbow flexion
C7	Radial	Triceps	Elbow extension
C7	Radial	Extensor digitorum	Finger extension
C8	Median and ulnar	Flexor digitorum	Finger flexion at MCP joint
T1	Median	Abductor pollicis brevis	Abduction of the thumb

Grading of power using the MRC scale

- 5 normal power
- 4 movement against resistance but not full power
- 3 movement against gravity but not resistance
- 2 movement with gravity removed
- 1 flicker of movement
- 0 no movement.

Reflexes

Assess the following reflexes:

- Biceps – with the arm relaxed and extended, tap the biceps tendon.
- Triceps – tap the triceps tendon with arm in flexed position
- Supinator – tap the radial tuberosity and look for pronation of the forearm.

Reflex root values	
Biceps	C5, C6
Triceps	C7
Supinator	C5

Coordination

- Tell the patient to rapidly pronate and supinate one hand on the back of the other. Demonstrate this to the patient first. Any abnormality indicates cerebellar disease.

- Tell the patient to touch their nose using a finger, and touch the examiner's finger which is placed at a reasonable distance in front of the patient. Look for an intention tremor and past-pointing, both indicating cerebellar disease.

Finishing off

- Thank the patient
- Make sure patient is comfortable and offer to help cover them up
- Wash hands
- Present and consider age of patient in forming differential
- Summarise.

Case presentation

"On examination, this patient has increased tone on the left hand side, with weakness. This is in a pyramidal distribution, with flexion stronger than extension. He also has increased reflexes with a brisk triceps reflex on the left. This would be consistent with an upper motor neuron lesion and the commonest cause of this would be a stroke."

Summary

☐ Inspect for wasting, fasciculation, tremor.

☐ Assess tone by rolling leg and lifting leg off the bed at the knee.

☐ If there is increased tone, check for the presence of ankle clonus.

☐ Test power: hip flexion, hip extension, knee flexion, knee extension, foot dorsiflexion, foot plantar flexion, extension of the great toe.

☐ Check ankle, knee and plantar reflexes.

☐ Test coordination by performing the heel–shin test.

☐ Perform Romberg's test.

☐ Assess the gait.

Examiner's instruction

"Examine the motor neurological system in the legs of this patient and present your findings."

General inspection

Stand at the end of the bed and look at the patient

- Muscle wasting
- Fasciculations
- Deformities/posture
- Tremor
- Wheelchair/walking stick
- Catheter
- Posture – is the patient hemiplegic?

Definitions

- **Clonus:** rapid involuntary muscular contraction upon sudden stretching of the muscle, associated with upper motor neuron lesion. Sustained clonus (3 beats or more) is considered abnormal.

- **Fasiculations:** local, involuntary muscle contractions, which can be seen under the skin.

- **Spasticity:** increased muscle tone associated with upper motor neuron lesions.

- **Hemiparesis:** weakness affecting the arm and leg on the same side of the body. Usually this results from a lesion in the internal capsule.

- **Paraparesis:** weakness affecting both legs. Usually caused by lesion in the spinal cord.

- **Tetraparesis:** weakness affecting all four limbs.

Tone

- Assess tone by:
  - rolling the each leg side to side
  - lifting the leg of the bed at the knee joint noting if the heel is lifted of the bed.

ACE TIP

Ask the patient if they are in any pain before you touch them

- Clonus – test this by rapidly dorsiflexing the ankle and noting the number the beats. More than three beats is abnormal and a sign of an upper motor neuron lesion.

> **Causes of spastic legs (the age of the patient may guide you)**
>
> - **Multiple sclerosis:** often in the younger patient
> - **Trauma:** look for scars
> - **Cord compression:** look for signs of malignancy, e.g., cachexia, radiotherapy tattoos
> - **Motor neuron disease:** may be flacci

Power

Assess power in the following muscle groups:

- **Hip flexors** – ilopsoas: Ask patient to raise the leg of the bed and stop you from pushing down.
- **Hip extensors** – gluteus maximus: ask patient to stop you from lifting the leg of the bed.
- **Knee flexors** – hamstrings: ask patient to bend the knee and stop you from pulling the leg straight.
- **Knee extensors** – quadriceps: ask the patient to bend the knee and stop you from pushing it.
- **Ankle dorsiflexors** – tibialis anterior: ask the patient to press down into your hand at the soles of feet.
- **Ankle plantar flexors** – gastrocnemius and soleus: ask patient to point toes towards them and stop you pushing feet down.
- **Great toe flexion** – extensor hallucis longus: ask patient to push their big toe up against your resistance.

Grade power using the MRC scale.

Root	Nerve	Muscle group tested	Muscle action tested
L1, L2	Femoral	Iliopsoas	Hip flexion
L5 S1	Inferior gluteal	Gluteus maximus	Hip extension
S1	Sciatic	Hamstrings	Knee flexion
L3, L4	Femoral	Quadriceps	Knee extension
L4, L5	Peroneal	Tibialis anterior	Foot dorsiflexion
S1, S2	Common peronial	Gastrocnemius and soleus	Foot plantar flexion
L5	Tibial	Extensor hallucis longus	Extension of the great toe

Grading of power using the MRC scale

- 5   normal power
- 4   movement against resistance but not full power
- 3   movement against gravity but not resistance

- 2   movement with gravity removed
- 1   flicker of movement
- 0   no movement

Reflexes:
- Test the knee jerk by placing one hand under the knee and tapping the patella tendon with the tendon hammer in the other hand.
- Test the ankle jerk by dorsiflexing the ankle and tapping the Achilles tendon.
- Test the plantar reflex (upgoing great toe in upper motor neuron lesions).

Reflex root values	
Knee jerk	L3, L4
Ankle	S1, S2

Reinforcement

If the reflex is absent, repeat with reinforcement. Ask the patient to clench their teeth or bear down as you test.

ACE TIP

In patients whose limbs are symmetrically weak and wasted in the proximal muscle groups, but with preservation of tone and power distally, think of a proximal myopathy. Ask the patient to stand from the sitting position.

Causes of a proximal myopathy

- **Inherited:** muscular dystrophy (young)
- **Endocrine/metabollic:** diabetes, Cushing's syndrome, thyrotoxicosis, acromegaly, osteomalacia
- **Drugs:** corticosteroids, alcohol
- **Dermatomyositis/polymyositis**

ACE TIP

If the signs appear to affect a number of nerves, consider a mononeuritis multiplex.

Causes of mononeuritis multiplex

- Diabetic neuropathy
- Connective tissue disorders (e.g., rheumatoid arthritis)
- Systemic lupus erythematosus
- Amyloidosis

Coordination

- Heel–shin test – ask the patient to use the heel of one foot and slide it along the opposite leg and raise the foot of the leg as fast as possible. Look for an intention tremor and uncoordination, which indicate cerebellar disease.

Gait

- Ask the patient to walk across the room and look for any abnormality of stance, and speed of gait. Look for antalgia, spacing of feet and any unsteadiness.

Abnormal gaits

- **Spastic gait:** the hemiplegic patient will have the characteristic flexed arm and extended leg with foot turned inwards, all on the same side of the body. The spastic leg is swung is swung in a circular fashion (circumduction) during walking. In the paraplegic patient, both feet are turned inwards and the action of the adductor muscles of the legs results in the so-called scissoring gait.

- **Parkinsonian gait:** the patient has a stooped posture, is slow to start walking, and the gait has a shuffling appearance with reduced swinging of the arms.

- **Cerebellar gait:** broad-based, unsteady gait. The patient sways from side to side (The "drunken sailor gait").

- **High stepping gait:** this is associated with foot drop, often due to common peroneal nerve palsy. The patient lifts the affected foot high off the ground.

- **Sensory ataxia:** the patient constantly looks at the ground while walking. The gait is broad-based and the feet stamp.

ACE TIPS

- If you suspect multiple sclerosis, offer to examine for cerebellar signs, internuclear ophthalmoplegia and to perform fundoscopy looking for optic atrophy.

- If you find the patient has spastic paraparesis, you must examine for a sensory level.

Finishing off

- Thank the patient
- Make sure patient is comfortable and offer to help cover them up
- Wash hands
- Present and consider age of patient in forming differential
- Summarise.

Case presentation

"On examination of this patient's legs, he has increased tone on the left side. He also has weakness of the left leg in a pyramidal distribution with extensors stronger than flexors. There are brisk reflexes, particularly at the knee on the left side. There is a hemiparetic, spastic gait. These signs are consistent with an upper motor neuron lesion, the commonest cause of which is a stroke."

Summary

☐ Patient comfortable with arms suitably exposed.

☐ Test sensation – light touch, pinprick, temperature, joint position, vibration.

Examiner's instruction:

"Examine the sensory neurological system in the arms of this patient and present your findings."

Wh Wash hands

I Introduce yourself and identify the patient

S Summarise what you are going to do

P Permission

E Exposure of patient. Expose the arms and trunk

R Reposition the patient

S State of patient – old/young, well/unwell.

General inspection

Stand at the end of the bed and look at the patient

- Muscle wasting of the arms. Observe from top to bottom – deltoids, biceps, triceps, interossei, thenar and hypothenar eminences
- Fasciculations
- Deformities, e.g., clawing of the hands
- Wrist drop.

ACE TIP

Ask the patient if they are in any pain before you touch them

---

At this stage, also palpate for any thickened nerves in the distribution of the median and ulnar nerves.

Instructing the patient

- It is important to inform the patient about the procedure for testing sensation.

- For each modality, first test the stimulus at the sternum with the patient's eyes open. If they can feel the stimulus at the sternum, instruct the patient to close their eyes and apply the stimulus at the areas to be tested.

- Instruct the patient to say "yes" when the stimulus is felt, and if it feels the same on both sides.

Apply the stimulus distally and move proximally noting the distribution and level of sensory loss. The distribution can be symmetrical in a glove distribution, or dermatomal. Always compare both sides.

Light touch

- Use a wisp of cotton wool to test light touch starting distally and moving proximally.

Key dermatomes in the arms

C4: shoulder

C5: lateral aspect of the arm

C6: lateral aspect of the forearm, thumb and index finer

C7: middle finger

C8: medial two fingers, medial aspect of the hand

T1: medial aspect of the forearm and elbow

T2: medial aspect of the upper arm

Pin-prick
- Use a neurotip or an orange stick to apply the stimulus distally moving proximally in each dermatome.

Temperature
- This modality is not tested often.
- Use a test tube or equivalent container with cold and warm water. Apply the stimuli in turn, asking the patient if the area of skin feels cold or warm, noting any difference in sensation.

Vibration sense
- Using a 128 Hz tuning fork, test vibration sense at bony prominences.
- Start by placing the tuning fork on the sternum to demonstrate the sensation.
- Instruct the patient to indicate when the sensation is felt and when it stops. Then place the tuning fork at bony prominences starting distally. Stop the vibration sense by placing your hand over the tuning fork. If no sensation is felt, place the tuning fork proximally until it is felt.
- Place the tuning fork at bony prominences starting distally and moving proximally if the sensation is not felt. In the upper limb, start at the finger tip, metacarpophalangeal joint, wrist, elbow and acromion.

Joint position sense (proprioception)
- Demonstrate to the patient what you are going to do. Using your thumb and index finger, hold the patient's index finger at the sides. Passively move the terminal phalanx, indicating to the patient which movement is up and down. Instruct the patient to close their eyes and tell you which way you are moving the joint. Start distally and move proximally if the initial movement is not felt.
- Start distally at the distal interphalangeal joint, and move proximally to the proximal interphalangeal joint, metacarpal–phalangeal joint, wrist, elbow and shoulder progressively if the initial movement is not sensed.

ACE TIP

If you find bilateral symmetrical loss of sensation, affecting all sensory modalities, think peripheral neuropathy. Weakness may or may not be present. Look for evidence of diabetes mellitus or chronic alcohol use.

ACE TIP

• **Proprioception** and **vibration** sensation travel in the dorsal column tracts

• **Temperature** and **pain** sensation travel in the spinothalamic tracts

Causes of a sensory peripheral neuropathy

• Diabetic neuropathy

• Alcohol

• B vitamin deficiency

• Chronic renal failure

Mononeuritis multiplex

Definition: an acute or subacute loss of sensory and motor function of individual peripheral nerves

Causes:

• Diabetic neuropathy

• Connective tissue disorders (e.g., rheumatoid arthritis)

• Systemic lupus erythematosus

• Amyloidosis

• Neoplasia

Finishing off

• Thank the patient

• Make sure patient is comfortable and offer to help cover them up

• Wash hands

• Present and consider age of patient in forming differential

• Summarise.

Also:

• Turn to the examiner and present clinical findings, stating which modalities are affected, the distribution and level of sensory loss.

• Tell the examiner that to finish of the examination you would like to perform the motor examination of the upper limbs, and perform the Phalen's and Tinnel's tests if you suspect carpal Tunnel syndrome.

• Give a list of differential diagnoses that are consistent with your findings.

Case presentation

"On examination of this patient's upper limbs, he has impairment of vibration sense to the wrists bilaterally. All other sensory modalities tested were preserved. This is consistent with pathology of the dorsal columns, sparing the spinothalamic tracts."

Neurology: Sensory Examination of the Legs

Summary

☐ Patient comfortable with legs suitably exposed.

☐ Test sensation: light touch, pinprick, temperature, joint position, vibration.

☐ Romberg's test and gait

Examiner's instruction

"Examine the sensory neurological system in the legs of this patient and present your findings."

Wh Wash hands

I Introduce yourself and identify the patient

S Summarise what you are going to do, e.g., "I would like to perform a series of tests to assess movement"

P Permission

E Exposure of patient – expose the legs up to the waist

R Reposition the patient

S State of patient (well/unwell).

General inspection

Stand at the end of the bed and look at the patient

- Muscle wasting of the legs in the major muscle groups
- Fasciculations of muscle groups
- Deformities, e.g., pes cavus
- Foot drop.

ACE TIPS

Ask the patient if they are in any pain before you touch them

Instructing the patient

- It is important to inform the patient about the procedure for testing sensation.

- For each modality, first test the stimulus at the sternum with the patient's eyes open. If they can feel the stimulus at the sternum, instruct the patient to close their eyes and apply the stimulus at the areas to be tested.

- Instruct the patient to say "yes" when the stimulus is felt, and if it feels the same on both sides.

ACE TIPS

- Remember to apply the stimulus distally and move proximally noting the distribution and level of sensory loss. The distribution can be symmetrical in a stocking distribution, or dermatomal.

- Always compare both sides.

Light touch

- Use a wisp of cotton wool to test light touch starting distally and moving proximally.

Key dermatomes in the legs

T10: Umbillicus

L1: Hip crease

L2: "Two hands in the pockets"

L3: is the knee

L5: **L**arge toe

S1: **S**mall toe

Pin-prick
• Use a neurotip or an orange stick to apply the stimulus distally moving proximally in each dermatome.

Temperature
• This modality is not tested often.

• Use a test tube or equivalent container with cold and warm water. Apply the stimulus in turn asking the patient if the area of skin feels cold or warm, noting any difference in sensation.

Vibration sense
• Using a 128 Hz tuning fork, test vibration sense at bony prominences.

• Start by placing the tuning fork on the sternum to demonstrate the sensation.

• Instruct the patient to indicate when the sensation is felt and when it stops. Then place the tuning fork at bony prominences starting distally. Stop the vibration sense by placing your hand over the tuning fork. If no sensation is felt, place the tuning fork proximally until it is felt.

ACE TIPS

Place the tuning fork at bony prominences starting distally and moving proximally if the sensation is not felt. In the lower limb, start at the first metatarsal phalangeal joint, medial malleolus, knee, and anterior superior iliac spine.

Joint position sense (proprioception)
• Demonstrate to the patient what you are going to do. Using your thumb and index finger, hold the patient's toe at the sides. Passively move the terminal phalanx, indicating to the patient which movement is up and down. Instruct the patient to close their eyes and tell you which way you are moving the joint. Start distally and move proximally if the initial movement is not felt.

ACE TIPS

Start distally at the distal interphalangeal joint, and move proximally to the metatarsal phalangeal joint, ankle and knee joints progressively if the initial movement is not sensed.

Be sure to hold the toe on the sides when you are moving it as holding on top and below the toe when moving it gives a pressure clue as to the direction you are moving the toe in and this doesn't test proprioception.

Romberg's test

- With the patient's eyes open, ask the patient to stand up with their feet together. Observe for unsteadiness. If the patient is unsteady with their eyes open, this indicates either vestibular or cerebellar dysfunction. This is not a positive Romberg's test, but indicates disturbance of balance.
- Then, only if the patient is not unsteady with their eyes open, instruct the patient to close their eyes and observe for unsteadiness. If the patient is unsteady with eyes closed, the Romberg's test is positive and this indicates impairment of joint proprioception.

Gait
- Assess gait by asking the patient to walk across the room and back observing for a high-stepping gait suggesting a foot drop, or a broad based gait with the patient looking down at his feet with stamping suggesting a dorsal column lesion.

Finishing off
- Thank the patient
- Make sure patient is comfortable and offer to help cover them up
- Wash hands
- Present and consider age of patient in forming differential
- Summarise.

Also:

- Turn to the examiner and present clinical findings, stating which modalities are affected, the distribution and level of sensory loss.
- Tell the examiner that to finish of the examination you would like to perform the motor examination of the lower limbs.
- Give a list of differential diagnoses that are consistent with your findings.

Case presentation
"On examination of this patient's lower limbs, there is a bilateral, symmetrical sensory loss in a stocking distribution, affecting the following modalities. There is loss of light touch to below the knees on both sides. There is loss of pin-prick to mid-shin level on both sides. There is loss of vibration sense to the ankles. Joint position sense and temperature were preserved. The most likely explanation for these signs is a peripheral neuropathy associated with diabetes mellitus."

Cranial Nerve Examination

Summary

☐ Patient sitting at the same eye level as examiner.

☐ Enquire about changes in sense of smell (I).

☐ Look at the patient for evidence of ptosis and deviation of eyes from the midline.

☐ Examine eye movements looking for abnormalities of movement and nystagmus. Ask about diplopia (III, IV, VI).

☐ Assess for rapid eye movements using thumb and fist technique.

☐ Test light touch and pin-prick in the three divisions of the trigeminal nerve on the face of the patient with their eyes closed (sensory branch of V).

☐ Ask patient to clench their teeth and then to open their mouth against your opposition (motor branch of V).

☐ Look at the patient's face for evidence of asymmetry. Test muscles of facial expression by asking patient to raise eyebrows, close eyes as tightly as possible against your opposition, blow out cheeks, smile, purse lips (VII).

☐ Inspect external auditory meatus for the vesicles of herpes zoster and ask about hearing and taste (VII).

☐ Test VIII nerve function informally by whispering into patient's ear. Perform Rinne's and Weber's tests (VIII).

☐ Ask patient to say "ahh" and inspect the palate and uvula for symmetrical elevation (IX, X). The gag reflex may be performed (not usually done).

☐ Ask patient to shrug their shoulders against your opposition. Ask patient to turn their head to one side against your opposition and then repeat in the other direction (XI).

☐ Examine tongue for wasting and fasiculation while it lies in the floor of the mouth. Ask patient to stick out their tongue and move it from side to side, noting any deviation (XII).

☐ Assess speech.

Examiner's instructions

"Examine this patient's cranial nerves. Please omit CNII from your examination."

"This lady complains of dribbling when she eats. Examine her cranial nerves and find out why."

Common OSCE cases

• Third nerve palsy
• Sixth nerve palsy
• Facial (VII) nerve palsy
• Bulbar and pseudobulbar palsies
• Nystagmus
• Horner's syndrome
• Ptosis
• Cerebellopontine angle syndrome

Key signs associated with common OSCE cases

• **Third nerve palsy:** unilateral ptosis, pupil dilated (surgical III), eye inferolaterally deviated (the "down and out" eye).

• **Facial nerve palsy:** unilaterally weak muscles of the face (facial asymmetry).

• **Bulbar palsy (LMN IX, X, XI and XII):** wasted, fasciculating tongue; dysarthria; dysphagia; drooling.

• **Pseudo-bulbar palsy (UMN IX, X, XI and XII):** spastic, small tongue; dysarthria ("hot potato" speech); dysphagia.

• **Nystagmus:** look for other cerebellar signs.

• **Horner' syndrome:** ptosis, miosis (constricted pupil); enophthalmos (sunken eye); anhydrosis; loss of sweating on face.

• **Cerebellar-pontine angle syndrome:** sensory loss in distribution of trigeminal nerve (V); facial weakness (VII); nystagmus; sensori-neural deafness (VIII) e.g., acoustic neuroma.

Wh Wash hands

I Introduce yourself and identify patient

S Summarise what you would like to examine

P Permission

E Equipment – neurology pin, cotton wool, tuning fork

R Reposition patient sitting on a chair at eye level with you, about one arms length away

S State of patient (well/unwell), look in particular for facial asymmetry, mouth or eyelid droop, pupil abnormalities, nasogastric tube

Signs around the bed – hearing aids, glasses, BM chart.

General inspection

Stand at the end of the bed and look at the patient

- Abnormalities of the eyes and head posture
- Abnormality of speech or voice
- General posture of the patient.

> **ACE TIPS**
>
> Ask the patient if they are in any pain before you touch them

I – Olfactory nerve

- Ask the patient if they have noticed any change in their sense of smell.

- With the patient's eyes closed, present the patient with coffee beans and orange peel, testing each nostril in turn.

II – Optic nerve

(covered in the eye station)

III, IV, VI – Oculomotor, trochlear and abducens

- Inspect for ptosis and any deviation of the eyes from the midline.

- Examine eye movements by asking the patient to follow your finger. Move your finger in an "H" shape looking for any abnormality of eye movement, and note the direction in which this occurs.

- Also look for nystagmus.

- Ask the patient if they have any double vision, and explore its details.

- Assess for rapid eye movements using alternating thumb and fist.

Eye movements and cranial nerve

- Superior rectus – upward movement (III)

- Inferior rectus – downward movement (III)

- Medial rectus – adducts (III)

- Lateral rectus – abducts (VI)

- Superior oblique – on adduction, downward movement (IV)

- Inferior oblique – on adduction, upward movement (III)

Definitions

Nystagmus: rhythmic oscillation of the eyes, sustained for more than a few beats. It can occur in a horizontal or vertical direction.

Ptosis: sagging or droopiness of the upper eyelid.

> **Causes of IIIrd nerve palsies**
>
> * IIIrd nerve palsies sparing the pupil – diabetes (mononeuritis monoplex), midbrain stroke, demyelination.
>
> * IIIrd nerve palsies with dilated pupil – "surgical IIIrd" i.e., compression of the IIIrd nerve e.g., from a posterior communicating aneurysm. This is because parasympathetic nerves (innervating the pupillary sphincter) are found on the outside of the IIIrd nerve.

> **Causes of ptosis**
>
> * Third nerve palsy – complete ptosis, dilated pupil, in a "down and out" position
>
> * Horner's syndrome – partial ptosis, small pupil
>
> * Myotonic dystrophy – Bilateral ptosis, myotonic facies
>
> * Myasthenia gravis – the ptosis is fatigable.

V – Trigeminal nerve

* Test the sensory component of this nerve – test light touch and pin-prick using cotton wool and an orange stick respectively. Ask the patient to close their eyes and tell you when they can feel the sensation and if it feels the same on both sides. Place the testing modality close to the midline on both sides in the dermatomes of the ophthalmic, maxillary and mandibular branches of the trigeminal nerve.

* Test the motor function of the trigeminal nerve by asking the patient to clench their teeth and palpating over the masseter muscles on both sides. Ask the patient to open their mouth and stop you from closing it.

* Test the corneal reflex by touching the cornea of the eyes using a wisp of cotton wool (note: if the patient is wearing contact lenses, you won't be able to perform corneal reflex, so ask them first).

* Test the jaw reflex by asking the patient to open their mouth a little and tap your finger placed over their chin.

VII – Facial nerve

("face, ear, taste, tear")

* Look at the patient's face for any asymmetry especially of the nasolabial fold.
* Test the muscles of facial expression by asking the patient to:
  * Raise their eyebrows (assesses frontalis muscle)
  * Close their eyes as tight as possible (assesses orbicularis oculi muscle)
  * Blow out their cheeks and smile (assesses orbicularis oris and buccinator muscles)
  * Inspect the external auditory meatus for herpes zoster lesions (affects VIIth and VIIIth nerves)
  * Ask about hearing and taste.

Differentiate UMN and LMN VIIth nerve

• Sparing of the upper face is an UMN sign.

• Involvement of the upper and lower part of the face is a LMN sign.

Causes of facial weakness

• UMN cause – stroke, demyelination

• LMN cause – Bell's palsy, parotid swelling, varicella zoster infection (Ramsay Hunt syndrome)

VIII – Vestibulocochlear nerve

• Start by asking the patient to close their eyes. Standing behind the patient, whisper a number into the patient's ear and ask the patient to tell you in which ear they can hear the number and to repeat the number.

• Rinne's test – using a 512-Hz tuning fork, first place it in front of the ear (air conduction) and then on the mastoid process (bone conduction) and ask the patient in what position the sound was loudest. Repeat on both sides.

• Weber's test – place the tuning fork on the centre of the forehead and ask the patient if the sound is equal in both ears or more loud on one side and to indicate which side.

Describing Rinne's test

• Rinne's test assesses impairment of air conduction of sound.

• Normally, air conduction is better than bone conduction. If sound is louder when the fork is placed on the mastoid process than in front of the ear it suggests conductive deafness in that ear.

Describing Weber's test

• Weber's test assesses sensory neuronal conduction of sound.

• Normally, sound should be heard equally in both ears. If sound is heard louder in one ear it suggests the opposite ear has sensorineuronal deafness.

IX & X – Glossopharangeal and vagus nerves

• Ask the patient to stick out their tongue and using a tongue depressor ask the patient to say "ahh" and look for symmetrical elevation of the soft palate and uvula.

• Gag reflex. Not often done.

XI – Accessory nerve
- Ask the patient to shrug their shoulders and maintain this position whilst you push down. Note any loss of power (assesses the trapezius).
- Ask the patient to turn their head to one side and stop you from pushing it to the other side. (feel the bulk of the sternocleidomastoid muscle on the opposite side to which the patient's head is turned).

XII – Hypoglossal nerve
- Ask the patient to open their mouth, examine for tongue wasting and fasciculation while in the floor of the mouth.
- Ask patient to stick out their tongue. Note any deviation of the tongue.
- Ask the patient to move the tongue from side to side to assess for any weakness of movement.

Definitions

Pseudobulbar palsy: bilateral upper motor neuron lesions of cranial nerves IX, X, XI and XII. Presents with dysphagia (difficulty in swallowing), dysarthria ("hot potato speech"), small and spastic tongue with a brisk jaw jerk.

Bulbar palsy: bilateral lower motor neuron lesions of cranial nerves IX, X, XI and XII. Presents with dysphagia (difficulty in swallowing), difficulty in chewing, slurring of speech, tongue is wasted and fasciculates, dribbling of saliva, soft palate weakness – ask the patient to say "aah".

Causes of IX, X, XI and XII palsies

- Pseudobulbar palsy – stroke, motor neuron disease and demyelinating disorders

- Bulbar palsy – motor neuron disease, Guillain–Barré syndrome

---

Causes of cerebellopontine angle syndrome

- Acoustic neuroma, meningioma, glioma in pons

- Cerebellar tumours

- Infiltration of meninges by neoplastic or infective processes (e.g., tuberculosis)

Finishing off
- Thank the patient
- Make sure patient is comfortable and offer to help cover them up
- Wash hands
- Present and consider age of patient in forming differential
- Summarise.

Case presentation

"This patient has a complete palsy of the third cranial nerve, as evidenced by the presence of a dilated pupil, an inferolaterally deviated globe and ptosis."

"This patient has a palsy of the seventh cranial nerve of upper motor neuron type, as evidenced by a unilateral facial weakness that spares the upper face. The most likely aetiology is a stroke and I would like to examine the patient for evidence of upper motor neuron signs in the limbs."

Investigations

Investigations are directed by clinical findings.

IIIrd nerve palsy

- CT brain
- Urine dipstick for glucose
- Thyroid function tests
- ESR in older patients to exclude temporal arteritis.

VIth nerve palsy

- CT brain (VIth nerve palsy is a false localising sign in raised intracranial pressure)
- Urine dipstick for glucose
- Consider MRI of brain and CSF analysis in younger patients to exclude multiple sclerosis.

VIIth nerve palsy

- CT of brain
- Urine dipstick for glucose if upper motor neuron type
- The commonest cause of lower motor neuron type VIIth nerve palsy is Bell's palsy
- Consider MRI of brain if any suspicion of multiple sclerosis
- The differential diagnosis widens in cases of bilateral VIIth nerve palsies and includes sarcoidosis (chest X-ray and serum angiotensin converting enzyme (ACE) levels) and Guillain – Barré syndrome (CSF analysis shows very high protein) and myaesthenia gravis (edrophonium test, antibodies to acetylcholine receptors and electromyography).

Nystagmus

Initial investigations are those of a cerebellar syndrome:

- MRI of brain, visual evoked potentials and CSF analysis for oilgoclonal bands to exclude multiple sclerosis
- MRI of brain to exclude posterior fossa tumours
- CT of brain to exclude stroke
- Thyroid function tests.

Ptosis and Horner's syndrome

- CT of brain (stroke)
- MRI of brain (demyelination)
- Chest X-ray to exclude pancoast tumour.

Bulbar and pseudobulbar palsy

- CT of brain (stroke)
- Electromyography (fasciculations in motor neuron disease)
- Formal swallowing assessment.

Cerebellopontine angle syndrome

- MRI of brain (acoustic neuroma, meningioma, pontine glioma)
- Audiography
- CSF analysis.

Cerebellum Examination

Summary

☐ Inspect patient for stigmata of chronic liver disease, evidence of alcohol abuse, evidence of anti-epileptic medication and hypothyroidism.

☐ Test speech for evidence of dysarthria: "British constitution", "West Register Street" and "baby hippopotamus".

☐ Examine the upper limbs for tone.

☐ Perform the finger–nose test and assess for past-pointing and intention tremor.

☐ Try to elicit dysdiadochokinesis.

☐ Examine the lower limbs for tone.

☐ Perform the heel–shin test.

☐ Assess the patient's gait, looking for evidence of a wide-based gait. Test tandem-walking.

Examiner's instruction

"Examine this patient's cerebellar system and present your findings."

"This patient has a tremor. Please examine as appropriate."

"This patient presents with altered speech, please examine as appropriate."

Key signs associated with common OSCE cases

Cerebellar signs using the mnemonic RANDISH:

Rebound

Ataxia

Nystagmus

Dysdiadochokinesia

Intention tremor (and dysmetria)

Slurred speech

Hypotonia

Wh Wash hands

I Introduce yourself and identify patient

S Summarise that you would like to examine the patient's movements

P Permission

R Reposition patient lying at a 45-degree angle

S State of patient

Signs around bed – observe the bedside surroundings for clues to the functional status of the patient, e.g., walking aids, wheelchair, catheter.

General inspection

Stand at the end of the bed and look at the patient

- Scars
- Asymmetry
- Neurological signs which may suggest the aetiology of cerebellar dysfunction.

Clues on inspection

- Peripheral stigmata of chronic liver disease (alcohol abuse)

- Weight loss (paraneoplastic cerebellar syndrome, particular from lung carcinomas; cerebellar metastases)

- Gum hypertrophy (phenytoin use)

- Hypothyroidism

- Friedreich's ataxia (pes cavus, kyphoscoliosis, muscle wasting)

- Hearing aid (deafness may suggest a cerebellopontine angle tumour)

Cerebellum function

- Eye movements

- Posture

- Balance

- Locomotion

- Coordination of voluntary movement

- Motor learning

ACE TIPS

Ask the patient if they are in any pain before you touch them

Eyes

- Examine the eyes for nystagmus. Ask the patient to follow your finger up, down, left and right.
- Examine saccadic eye movements in both the horizontal and vertical planes.
- Ask the patient to look from one target to another (e.g., from your right hand to your left hand). Observe the eyes for hypometric saccades.

> **Definitions**
>
> **Nystagmus:** rhythmic oscillation of the eyes, sustained for more than a few beats. It can occur in a horizontal or vertical direction.
>
> **Hypometric saccades:** saccades are quick, simultaneous movements of both eyes in the same direction.
>
> **Dysarthria:** a speech disorder characterised by poor articulation of words or syllables.
>
> **Dysmetria:** past pointing
>
> **Dysdiadochokinesia:** abnormality in rapid alternating movements

Speech
- Ask the patient to repeat the following statements back to you and listen for dysarthria:
    - British constitution
    - West Register Street
    - Baby hippopotamus.

Upper limbs
- Ask the patient to hold out their arms fully stretched in front of them with the palms facing upwards and then close their eyes.

    Gently push the arms down observing for overshoot. This is oscillation of the arms before returning to its original position and is called rebound.
- Examine the arms for hypotonia.
- Finger–nose test:

    Start by positioning your own finger in front of the patient so that the patient can comfortably stretch their arm to touch it. Ask the patient to use the index finger of their hand to first touch their nose then the examiner's finger as quickly as possible.

    Observe for intention tremor as the patient reaches out to touch the examiner's finger and for dysmetria – overshooting of the target.
- Elicit dysdiadochokinesia:

    Ask the patient to tap the palm of one hand on the back of the other then pronate and supinate the hand as quickly as possible. Perform the test on both sides.

Lower limbs
- Examine the legs for tone – looking for hypotonia.
- Heel–shin test:

    With the patient lying down, instruct the patient to use the heel of one foot to touch the opposite knee, slide the foot down the leg and lift up the foot to touch the examiner's hand, which should be positioned at a level above the patient's foot. Observe for incoordination of movement, an intention tremor and dysmetria.

- Gait – instruct the patient to:

    Walk across the room, walking alongside the patient at all times ensuring that the patient does not fall. Observe for a wide-based gait and the side on which the patient is unsteady.

    Tandem-walk, that is, ask the patient to walk as if they are walking along a tightrope, looking for ataxia. Note the side to which the patient falls.

Chronic causes of cerebellar syndrome

Hereditary:

- Spinocerebellar ataxias (Friedreich's ataxia)

Acquired:

• Inflammatory	Multiple sclerosis
• Neoplastic	Posterior fossa tumour
	Cerebellopontine angle tumour
	Paraneoplastic syndromes (lung carcinoma, breast, pelvic)
• Vascular	Stroke
• Drugs	Alcohol, anti-epileptics, particularly phenytoin
• Metabolic	Hypothyroidism
	Wilson's disease

Localize the cerebellar lesion accordingly to clinical findings

Lesions of the vermis are characterised by:

- Wide-based gait

- Inability to tandem walk

- Truncal ataxia, which is the inability to stand up without support

- Abnormal eye movements as evidenced by nystagmus, and jerky pursuits

Lesions of the cerebellar hemisphere are characterised by:

- Uncoordination of limb movements which is evidenced by an intention tremor, dysmetria and dysdiadochokinesia

- Staccato speech

Finishing off

- Thank the patient
- Make sure patient is comfortable and offer to help cover them up
- Wash hands
- Present and consider age of patient in forming differential
- Summarise.

Mention that you would like to:

- Perform the rest of the neurological examination (motor and sensory) and cranial nerve examination especially testing for V, VII and VIII function, assessing for signs of a cerebellopontine angle tumour.
- Perform fundoscopy looking for optic atrophy of multiple sclerosis.

Case presentation

"This patient has a cerebellar syndrome as evidenced by an ataxic gait, nystagmus, dysarthria and intention tremor. I would like to take a drug history, perform fundoscopy and do a complete neurological examination to identify the cause."

Investigations

- Full blood count (macrocytosis) and liver function tests may reveal evidence of alcohol abuse
- MRI of brain to look for tumour, abscess, infarction, haemorrhage and demyelination
- Thyroid function tests
- Monitoring of serum levels of anti-epileptic agents, if appropriate
- Investigations for lung and ovarian neoplasms (paraneoplastic cerebellar syndrome)
- Investigations for Wilson's disease.

Parkinsonism Examination

Summary

☐ Patient resting on bed, arms and legs exposed.

☐ Look at the patient for expressionless face (hypomimia), slow blinking of eyes, drooling and unilateral pill-rolling tremor.

☐ Assess tone in arms, with particular attention to the wrist. Look for rigidity and cog-wheeling at the wrist.

☐ Assess for bradykinesia – ask patient to touch each finger with their thumb.

☐ Assess eye movements looking for impaired vertical gaze.

☐ Perform the glabellar tap.

☐ Assess speech by asking the patient to say: "Today is Sunday and the sun is shining". Listen for slow, monotonous speech.

☐ Assess functional status – look at handwriting for micrographia. Ask patient to undo buttons, tie up shoes.

☐ Check gait – look for loss of arm swing, hesitation and freezing, difficulty turning round, stooped posture, small steps and shuffling gait.

Examiner's instructions

"This patient has an obvious tremor. Inspect the tremor and continue to examine the patient as appropriate."

"Observe this patient and examine as appropriate."

"This patient presents with a history of falls and difficulty walking, please examine as appropriate."

Listen to the instructions carefully. If the instruction states that the patient presents with a history of falls, begin by examining the gait first. If you notice the characteristic gait of parkinsonism, state this and proceed to demonstrate other signs of parkinsonism. Likewise, if the instruction tells you that the patient has a tremor, begin by demonstrating the type of tremor and proceed to elicit other signs of parkinsonism.

Wh Wash hands

I Introduce yourself and identify the patient

S Summarise what you are going to do, e.g., "I would like to perform a series of tests to assess movement"

P Permission

E Exposure of patient – expose the arms and legs

R Reposition the patient

S State of patient (well/unwell)

Signs around bed – walking sticks, Zimmer/Rolator frames.

Features of parkinsonism

Mnemonic TRAMESS:

Tremor

Rigidity

Akinesia/bradykinesia

Micrographia

Eye movements (glabellar tap and impaired upward gaze in supranuclear palsy)

Speech – slow and monotonous

Shuffling gait – stooped posture decreased arm swing

General inspection

Stand at the end of the bed and look at the patient

- Expressionless face – a very characteristic facial appearance also known as hypomimia
- Slow movements – infrequent blinking of the eyes
- Drooling
- Speech – ask the patient some questions, or during introduction, note slowing of speech or the staccato speech of cerebellar disease
- Posture – forward flexion
- Resting tremor – characteristic unilateral pill-rolling tremor (circular movement of thumb and index finger. In addition some patients also exhibit pronation and supination of the forearm). The tremor is most evident in the hands, but can also be noted at other sites, therefore look at the legs and jaw at rest.

> ### Definition
>
> **Parkinson's disease:** a chronic, slowly-progressive disorder caused by loss of dopaminergic neurons in the substantia nigra.

> ### ACE TIPS
>
> Ask the patient if they are in any pain before you touch them

Hands and arms

- Resting tremor (4–6 Hz) – if the tremor is not particularly evident, induce the tremor by distracting the patient by instructing the patient to either (a) close their eyes and count backwards from 100, or (b) tap their knee using the other hand, and observe the resting hand for a tremor.
- Rigidity – assess the tone in the arms, paying particular attention to tone at the wrist. Note rigidity (and the superimposed tremor),which is termed leadpipe rigidity. There may be cog-wheeling at the wrist.
- Bradykinesia – instruct the patient to use their thumb to touch each of their fingers in the same hand as fast as possible. Observe the action for slowing of the movement and reduction in the amplitude of movement. The latter is termed hypokinesia.

Face

- Assess eye movements to determine any impairment in vertical gaze (a feature of progressive supranuclear palsy, a Parkinson plus syndrome).
- Glabellar tap – tap the forehead of the patient between the eyebrows to demonstrate Myerson's sign. The sign is negative if the patient ceases to blink with tapping; this is normal. A positive sign is demonstrated by continued blinking upon tapping of the forehead. This is a primitive reflex and not a reliable test.
- Speech – ask the patient to say: "Today is Sunday and the sun is shining". Listen for slow, monotonous speech.

Functional status

Assess the degree of functional impairment due to disease by:

- Assessing handwriting – micrographia
- Assessing ability to undo buttons, tie up shoe laces, stand from a seated position.

Gait

- Ask the patient to walk across the room, turn around as quickly as possible and walk back. Observe for the following:
- Asymmetrical loss of arm swing
- Difficulty initiating gait (hesitation) and freezing
- Difficulty turning around
- Stooped posture

> ### ACE TIP
>
> The diagnosis of parkinsonism is clinical. It is important to exclude the Parkinson plus syndromes by appropriate investigations. In a young patient presenting with parkinsonian symptoms, always investigate for Wilson's disease.

- Small steps.
- Shuffling gait.

Causes of parkinsonism	
• Idiopathic:	Parkinson's disease
• Drug induced:	Neuroleptics (e.g., haloperidol, chlorpromazine) Antiemetics (e.g., metoclopramide)
• Toxins:	Heavy metal poisoning MPTP (by-product of heroin synthesis) Carbon monoxide poisoning
• Vascular:	Basal ganglia ischaemia
• Parkinson plus syndromes:	Multisystem atrophy (MSA) Progressive supranuclear palsy (PSP) Dementia with Lewy bodies (DLB) Cortical basal dementia (CBD)

Finishing off
- Thank the patient
- Make sure patient is comfortable and offer to help cover them up
- Wash hands
- Present and consider age of patient in forming differential
- Summarise.

Mention that you would:
- Measure lying and standing blood pressure noting a postural drop (postural hypotension is a feature of multisystem atrophy).
- Examine the drug chart.

Case presentation
"This patient has parkinsonism as evidenced by an expressionless face. He/she has an asymmetrical resting tremor, bradykinesia and leadpipe rigidity. He also has a typical gait of parkinsonism, with a stooped posture and a slow, shuffling gait."

Investigations
Parkinson's disease is essentially a clinical diagnosis.

⬤ Tremor Examination

Examiner's instructions

"Examine the tremor in this patient and present your findings."

The examiner's instruction is often misinterpreted. Many students tend to think that the diagnosis has already been given to them and thus focus on demonstration of the tremor by focussing on examination of the hands only.

Tremor is a symptom of an underlying disease process; therefore, the demonstration of the tremor is only part of what is required in this station. It is important to examine other areas to identify the cause of the tremor.

In order to do this successfully, it is important to have a classification of tremor in mind and a list of causes of a tremor to facilitate a thorough examination. This is outlined in the sections that follow.

Common OSCE cases

• Resting tremor as part of parkinsonism
• Intention tremor as part of cerebellar syndrome
• Postural tremor

In this scenario the examiner will want you to exclude the other causes of a tremor.

Definition

Tremor: a rhythmic oscillatory movement disorder that can affect any part of the body.

Key features of common OSCE cases

• Resting tremor (parkinsonism):

Mnemonic TRAMESS

Tremor

Rigidity

Akinesia/ bradykinesia

Micrographia

Eye movements (glabellar tap and impaired upward gaze in supranuclear palsy)

Speech – slow and monotonous

Shuffling gait – stooped posture decreased arm swing

• Intention tremor (cerebellar syndrome):

Key features of common OSCE cases—cont'd

Mnemonic RANDISH

Rebound

Ataxia

Nystagmus

Dysdiadochokinesia

Intention tremor (and dysmetria)

Slurred speech

Hypotonia

* Postural tremor (multiple associations)

  Signs of thyrotoxicosis, alcohol abuse, family history, drug history (β-agonists)

Wh   Wash hands

I   Introduce yourself and identify the patient

S   Summarise what you are going to do, e.g., "I would like to perform a series of tests to examine the cause of your tremor"

P   Permission

E   Exposure of patient – expose the arms and legs

R   Reposition the patient

S   State of patient (well/unwell).

General inspection

Stand at the end of the bed and look at the patient

* **Head:** titubation (nodding of the head), which occurs in benign essential tremor
* **Face:** the expressionless "mask-like facies" of parkinsonism may be apparent. Also look for features of tardive dyskinesia secondary to long term use of neuroleptics, i.e., dystonia and tics. A jaw tremor may be present in Parkinson's disease (PD)
* **Eyes:** signs of thyroid eye disease, reduced blink rate of PD
* **Neck:** swelling (goitre)
* **Arms and hands:** inspect for a resting tremor of parkinsonism and for dystonia
* **Trunk and legs:** look for a tremor at other sites.

ACE TIP

A unilateral resting tremor is characteristic of parkinsonism. A bilateral postural tremor is characteristic of benign essential tremor.

> ### Classification of tremors
>
> The simplest way to classify tremors is the relationship to voluntary movement:
>
> * Resting (the tremor is present at rest): parkinsonism
>
> * Intention (the tremor is only present during movement): cerebellar syndrome
>
> * Postural (the tremor is present during maintenance of a posture, e.g., holding the hands outstretched):
>
>   Benign essential tremor (improved by alcohol)
>
>   Thyrotoxicosis
>
>   Alcohol
>
>   Drugs, e.g., salbutamol, caffeine, lithium
>
>   Drug withdrawal syndromes, e.g., benzodiazepines

Hands

* Resting tremor – if no tremor was observed on inspection, one can try to elicit a resting tremor by distracting the patient by either (a) asking the patient to close their eyes and count backwards from 100, or (b) asking the patient to tap their knee with one hand whilst observing the resting hand for a tremor. If present, indicates you should look for other signs of parkinsonism.

* Intention tremor – perform finger–nose test. Instruct the patient to fully stretch out their arms in front of them, this time with palms facing up, and ask the patient to close their eyes and gently push the hand down. Note overshoot, i.e., does the hand oscillate before returning to its original position? This is called the rebound phenomenon. If present, proceed to examine cerebellar function.

* Postural tremor – instruct the patient to flex the elbow with the hands fully extended and abduct the shoulder, looking for a bilateral postural tremor in this position (implies a benign essential tremor). Instruct the patient to fully stretch out their arms in front of them with palms facing down. Place a piece of paper across the hands to look for a fine tremor. If this is present, go on to examine for signs of thyroid disease and chronic liver disease, and ask to see the drug chart.

Gait

Instruct the patient to walk across the room observing for:

* Shuffling gait indicative of parkinsonism
* Ataxia and impaired tandem gait suggesting cerebellar disease.

> ### ACE TIP
>
> If a resting tremor is present, proceed to examine the patient to demonstrate other features of parkinsonism and, likewise, if an intention tremor is present, continue the examination to demonstrate signs of cerebellar dysfunction.

Assess functional status

Once a tremor has been demonstrated, assess the functional status by asking the patient to perform several tasks:

- Write a sentence
- Draw a spiral
- Pick up an object
- Hold a glass of water.

Finishing off

- Thank the patient
- Make sure patient is comfortable and offer to help cover them up
- Wash hands
- Present and consider age of patient in forming differential
- Summarise.

Case presentation

"This patient has a resting tremor that would be consistent with a diagnosis of parkinsonism. I would like to examine him/ her further for evidence of parkinsonism."

Investigations

Intention tremor

Investigations are those of a cerebellar syndrome:

- Multiple sclerosis – MRI of brain, visual evoked potentials, CSF analysis (oligoclonal bands)
- Posterior fossa tumours – MRI of brain
- Hypothyroidism – thyroid function tests
- Stroke – CT of brain.

Postural tremor

- Thyroid function tests.

Resting tremor

- Parkinson's is essentially a clinical diagnosis.

● Speech Examination

Examiner's instruction

"Ask this patient some questions and proceed as appropriate."

"Please examine this patient's speech."

ACE TIP

By far the most commonest case in the examination is a patient with cerebellar dysarthria.

The three types of speech disturbance

Aphasia: difficulty with comprehension or formulation of language

Dysarthria: impaired articulation of speech

Dysphonia: impaired voice production

Wh Wash hands

I   Introduce yourself and identify the patient

S   Summarise what you are going to do, e.g., "I would like to perform a series of tests to assess your speech"

P   Permission

E   Exposure of patient

R   Reposition the patient

S   State of patient (well/unwell).

General inspection

Stand at the end of the bed and look at the patient

Observe the patient, looking for other neurological signs, which may give clues regarding the aetiology of the altered speech:

- Rest tremor would suggest parkinsonism
- Intention tremor would suggest cerebellar syndrome
- Patient with a hemiparesis would suggest a stroke.

Testing for Aphasia

- Assess fluency of speech – ask the patient some simple questions, e.g., "What is your full name and address?" Does the patient use words correctly?

- Assess comprehension of speech – give a simple command, e.g., "Close your eyes". If successful, try a more complicated three-step command, e.g., "Take this piece of paper in your right hand, fold it in half and place it on your left knee".
- Assess for word finding difficulties – ask the patient to name objects, e.g., watch, watch strap, buckle, and pen.
- Assess for repetition – ask the patient to repeat a simple phrase, e.g., "No ifs, ands or buts". If successful try more complicated phrases.

Definition of aphasia/dysphasia

Aphasia/dysphasia (these two words are commonly interchangeable) – results from damage to the speech centres. In most individuals the left cerebral hemisphere is dominant for language function, except in a minority of left-handed people who are right hemisphere dominant. There are two main types of aphasia: receptive and expressive (see below).

- **Receptive aphasia or sensory aphasia** – patients have impaired comprehension and cannot follow a simple command. The speech output is fluent but meaningless as the words are often wrong or jumbled up. If the patient uses incorrect words, this is termed "verbal paraphasia". However, the use of a meaningless word is termed "jargon aphasia". Receptive aphasia results from lesions in the Wernicke's area, which lies on the posterior section of the superior temporal gyrus in the dominant hemisphere.

- **Expressive aphasia or motor aphasia** – patients have preserved comprehension and can successfully follow commands. The speech output is non-fluent with word finding difficulties. The patient is often aware of their speech deficit and finds it very frustrating. There is usually an associated agraphia (inability to express thoughts in writing). Expressive aphasia results from lesions in the Broca's area, which lies on the posterior section of the inferior frontal gyrus of the dominant hemisphere.

Other patterns of aphasia

- **Global aphasia** – this describes a mixed picture with deficits in both speech comprehension and expression. Global aphasia results form large lesions involving both Broca's and Wernicke's areas. The commonest cause of this would be an ischaemic stroke.

- **Conduction aphasia** – characteristically patients have impaired repetition and this results from lesions in the arcuate fasciculus, which links the Wernicke's area to the Broca's area.

- **Nominal aphasia** – difficulty naming objects even though the patient knows what they are. Nominal aphasia results from lesions in the angular gyrus and does not commonly occur on its own but usually as part of a wider aphasia.

Testing for dysphonia

- Assess the quality of the speech – is the patient able to produce normal volume speech?
- Ask the patient to cough – listen to the quality of the cough e.g. is it a bovine cough?

Definition of dysphonia

Dysphonia results due to either paralysis of the vocal cords or due to structural disease of the larynx, e.g., laryngitis or tumour. Vocal cord paralysis produces quiet speech, almost a whisper. In addition the cough is weak. Rather than having an explosive quality at onset produced by sudden opening of the larynx, in patients with impaired laryngeal function the cough is described as "bovine" as it lacks the explosive quality. Neurological causes include:

- Myasthenic weakness affecting the laryngeal muscles

- Focal mononeuropathy affecting the laryngeal nerve

- Polyneuropathy affecting the laryngeal nerves, e.g., Guillain-Barré syndrome

- Motor neurone disease affecting the vagus motor neuron

- Focal lesions compressing the recurrent laryngeal nerve, e.g., Pancoast's syndrome.

Note: dysphonia can be non-organic and in these cases the cough is normal (this is not likely to appear in the examination).

ACE TIPS

- Dysphonia with a normal cough implies a laryngeal lesion

- Dysphonia with a bovine cough implies vocal cord palsy

Testing for dysarthria

- Listen for slurred, staccato speech – ask the patient to say "West Register Street", "baby hippopotamus" or even "British constitution".
- Ask the patient to say ma, ma, ma then la, la, la, then, ca, ca, ca, followed by ga, ga, ga. This will help to assess the area that is affected (difficulty with ma = impaired lip movements; difficulty with la = impaired tongue movements; difficulty with ca = impaired movement of soft palate; and difficulty with ga = impaired movement of lower pharynx).
- Examine the patient's mouth – look at the tongue and observe for wasting or fasciculation. Assess palatal movements and note if they are symmetrical.
- Elicit the jaw jerk and suggest that you would want to perform the gag reflex for completeness (but do not perform this).

Definition of dysarthria

Dysarthria results due to a disorder in speech articulation. Normal articulation depends on successful coordination of breathing, vocal cords, larynx, pharynx, lips and tongue. Common types of dysarthria are listed below:

- **Spastic (pseudobulbar palsy)** – slow monotonous speech, often described as "hot potato speech". Other signs are a spastic immobile tongue, brisk jaw jerk, brisk gag reflex, the patient is emotionally labile and in addition there are often associated upper motor neuron signs in the limbs. Spastic dysarthria results from bilateral upper motor neurone weakness and a common cause of this is bi-hemispheric vascular disease.

- **Cerebellar** – slurred, scanning speech (each syllable in a word receives equal stress) and a disordered speech rhythm. A common cause is multiple sclerosis.

- **Extrapyramidal** – quiet, monotonous speech.

- **Lower motor neuron, nerve or muscle lesions (bulbar palsy)** – difficulty with certain sounds depends on which muscle group has been affected, e.g., palatal weakness (Xth cranial nerve lesion) causes nasal speech and in particular the patient has difficulty with the sound "ca", tongue weakness (XIIth cranial nerve lesion) causes distorted speech and difficulty with the sound "la" and facial weakness (VIIth cranial nerve lesion) causes difficulty with the sound "ma". Other signs consistent with a bulbar palsy are an absent jaw jerk, reduced or absent gag reflex and wasted fasciculating tongue. There may also be dysphagia and nasal regurgitation present. Possible causes include, motor neurone disease or Guillain-Barré syndrome.

Finishing off
- Thank the patient
- Make sure patient is comfortable and offer to help cover them up
- Wash hands
- Present and consider age of patient in forming differential
- Summarise.

Mention that you would like to
- Examine the rest of the cranial nerves in particular assessing for impairment of cranial nerves IX–XII (if you suspect a bulbar palsy).
- Examine other facets of language, e.g., reading and writing (if you suspect a dysphasia).
- Test for other signs compatible with a cerebellar syndrome, e.g., intention tremor and nystagmus (if you suspect a cerebellar syndrome).

Eye Examination

Summary

☐ Patient sitting on chair.

☐ Inspect for ptosis, position of pupils and size of pupils.

☐ Assess visual acuity either informally (e.g., by reading newsprint) or formally with a Snellen chart.

☐ Examine visual fields by confrontation, comparing the patient's visual fields with your own.

☐ Assess colour vision using the Ishihara chart (not usually required in the exam, but offer to do it).

☐ Test pupillary reaction to light (looking for a relative afferent pupillary defect) and accommodation.

☐ Perform fundoscopy.

Examiner instructions

"Examine this patient's eyes."

"This gentleman has double vision. Examine his eyes and find the cause."

"Examine this patient's fundi and describe any abnormalities."

Common OSCE cases
- Horner's syndrome and ptosis
- Cranial nerve palsies
- Visual field defects
- Nystagmus.

Key signs of common OSCE cases

- **Horner's syndrome:** ptosis, miosis (constricted pupil), enophthalmos (sunken eye), anhydrosis (loss of sweating on face)

- **Third nerve palsy:** unilateral ptosis, pupil dilated (surgical III), eye inferomedially deviated (the "down and out" eye)

- **Sixth nerve palsy:** eye deviated medially with failure of abduction

- **Visual field defects:** central scotoma; homonymous hemianopia: bitemporal hemianopia

- **Nystagmus:** usually horizontal nystagmus +/– cerebellar signs

---

Wh Wash hands
I Introduce yourself and identify patient
S Summarise that you would like to examine the patients eyes
P Permission
E Equipment – Snellen chart, 10 mm red hat pin, ophthalmoscope
R Reposition patient sitting on a chair
S State of patient (well/unwell)
Signs around bed – eye drops, glasses, drugs e.g. antihypertensives, diabetic medication

General inspection

Stand at the end of the bed and look at the patient

Assess:
- Ptosis
- Position
- Pupil size.

> **Causes of Horner's syndrome**
>
> - Lesion in the brain stem – demyelination or stroke (as part of lateral medullary syndrome)
> - Lesion in the cord – syringomyelia
> - Lesion in the neck – apical lung cancer (Pancoast's tumour), aneurysm

> **Diagnosis on inspection of pupils**
>
> - **Horner's syndrome:** ptosis, miosis, anhidrosis, enophthalmos
> - **Argyll Robertson pupil:** accommodation retained light lost
> - **Third nerve palsy:** fixed, dilated pupil; eye looks "down and out"; ptosis
> - **Holmes Adie pupil (myotonic pupil):** one pupil more dilated than the other; common in young women

Visual acuity

"I'd like to measure how much you can see of this chart from this distance. Please read out the letters from the top downwards as far as you can."

- Reposition patient 6 metres away from Snellen chart.
- Unaided assessment – remove glasses/contact lenses, however, you may want measurements with glasses on also.
- Ask patient to cover one eye and read down from the top of chart:
  - Record the lowest line read correctly
  - Findings – patient could only read 3/5 letters on 5th line correctly
  - Interpretation – a normal eye can read the 5th line up to 12 metres away (as indicated on Snellen chart); there were two errors made whilst reading the fifth line
  - Recording – (6/12) – 2
  - Numerator – distance (m) from which chart is read
  - Denominator – the maximum distance (m) a normal eye could read the lowest line read correctly
  - –x – the number of errors made whilst reading the lowest line.
- Repeat this with other eye.
- If patient cannot read the first line, bring them 3 m/2 m/1 m from chart.
- If patient cannot read top line at 1 m distance from chart, can they, at 0.5 m, count fingers, perceive hand movements, differentiate between light and dark.

Visual fields

- Examine by confrontation – compare patient's visual field to examiner's, assuming examiner's is normal.

- Reposition patient sitting on a chair 1 metre away from you at eye level.
- Test left eye – "Could you kindly cover your right eye with your right hand and look at the bridge of my nose. Without actually looking at my hands, can you tell me when you can see my finger?"
- Cover your left eye with left hand.
- Beginning in the periphery, bring a moving finger from right hand toward the centre.
- Ask patient to respond when moving finger is first seen.
- Repeat as if travelling along the spokes of a wheel, testing upper and lower temporal zones.
- Cover your left eye with right hand. Use moving finger from left hand to examine patient's nasal field.
- Use opposite hands to test the other eye.

Causes of visual field abnormalities

Central scotoma: maculopathy or damage to the optic nerve giving central vision disturbance

Bitemporal hemianopia: lesion at the optic chiasm, usually involving the pituitary gland; look for stigmata of acromegaly or pituitary insufficiency

Homonymous hemianopia: usually caused by a middle cerebral artery (MCA) stroke; a right MCA lesion will cause a left homonymous hemianopia and vice versa

Homonymous quadrantanopia: lesion in the temporal radiations

Colour vision
- Use Ishihara chart – often not necessary in exam, but offer it.

Pupillary reaction to light
- Shine a torch beam into the pupil from the side – do not shine it straight in front of the eye as the pupil may constrict due to accommodation of the near object.
  - Look for pupillary constriction (direct light response).
  - Look again in the opposite eye (consensual light response).
  - Repeat method in opposite eye.
- Swinging light reflex – look for relative afferent papillary defect (RAPD). This can occur in any damage to the retina that prevents it from detecting light and activating the parasympathetic response to pupil constriction, e.g., optic neuritis (MS), optic atrophy.
  - Shine light into the good eye, this will constrict both pupils as there is both direct and consensual response.
  - When you swing light into the bad eye the both pupils dilate as light cannot stimulate the parasympathetic pupil constriction.
  - On returning light into the good eye both pupils constrict.
  - *So, essentially, direct is lost and consensual remains.*

Pupillary reaction to accommodation
• Ask patient to focus on a distant point.

• Bring your finger to about 15 cm away and ask patient to focus on finger.

• Look for pupillary constriction.

Eye movements
• Hold one finger about 30–40 cm away from their face. Move your finger to each side, asking about double vision and looking for nystagmus.

Causes of ptosis

Unilateral: third cranial nerve palsy; Horner's syndrome

Bilateral: myasthenia gravis; myotonic dystrophy (look at the face); congenital; bilateral third cranial nerve palsies

---

ACE TIP

The slow beat of nystagmus is the abnormal one as the fast beat is the brain's way of trying to correct the abnormal eye movement. Causes of horizontal nystagmus can seem complicated but try and distinguish:

• Cerebellar (slow beat towards side of lesion)

• Vestibular (slow beat away from side of lesion)

• Brainstem (could be either)

ACE TIP

If the patient can see double on a particular movement, e.g., lateral gaze to the left, try and establish in which eye the problem is. You can do this by asking the patient to shut each eye in turn when looking in the direction that causes double vision. Whichever eye, when shut, removes the lateral of the two images, is the abnormal eye and there may be a muscle/nerve problem in that eye.

Fundoscopy

ACE TIP

The image of the back of the eye seen using an ophthalmoscope is known as the fundus. Students fear they need a detailed understanding of ophthalmology to interpret fundal images and worry how they may achieve this, with such little time devoted to ophthalmology during their MBBS training. The truth is, the most important image of the fundus to get to grips with is that of the normal fundus as there are only a limited number of abnormalities that you are likely to see and most are listed below.

- Make sure you are in a dark room and comment on using tropicamide ideally to dilate the pupil.
- Use your right eye and right hand to look at their right eye.
- Start about 1.5 m away and elicit the red reflex. Then move in slowly from an angle of 45 degrees from the temporal side – this way the optic disc should come into view without much searching.

Optic disk

- Focus on the blood vessels on the retina and follow them to the optic disk where they all meet.
- Look at each quadrant of the retina.

Comment on the colour

- Red – normal
- Pale – optic atrophy.

Comment on the margin of the optic disk

- Defined (you can see an obvious circle outlining the optic disk) – normal
- Blurred – papilloedema.

Comment on the cup:disk ratio

Blood vessels travelling along the plane of the retina dip perpendicularly through the centre of the optic disk to exit the eye. The dipping of the vessels through the disk creates the appearance of a circle within the disk, known as the optic cup. The normal cup:disk ratio is about 0.3. Atrophy of the nerves in the disk (glaucomatous change) results in the vessels exiting through the periphery of the disk. As the vessels dip in the periphery, the cup appears larger. You can describe this as an increased cup:disk ratio – this is the sign of glaucoma.

Two sets of blood vessels appear to curve out from the disk towards the temporal side of the fundus. *Identify the superior curve (upper) and inferior curve (lower)* – these are known as arcades.

There are both arterioles and veins within these arcades. The arterioles are redder and narrower than the veins.

Comment on the arteries

- Normal
- Narrowed – hypertensive retinopathy (copper wiring)
- Arteriovenous nipping – here the less compliant artery forces the vein to go deeper into the retina, indicating diabetic hypertensive retinopathy
- Neovascularisation (new vessel formation) – proliferative diabetic retinopathy.

Comment on the veins

- Normal
- Venous dilations – central retinal vein obstruction, hypertensive retinopathy, papilloedema
- Venous loops – preproliferative diabetic retinopathy.

Macula

The macula is found two optic disk widths away from the temporal side of the optic disc and is viewed best by asking the patient to look directly at the light.

Comment on the appearance of the macula

* Orange/red – normal
* Pale – central retinal artery occlusion.

Look at each quadrant of the retina

* Microaneurysm – small red patches of dilated vessels secondary to hypertensive/background diabetic retinopathy
* Hard exudates – well-defined bright yellow clusters of fat deposited from vessels in background diabetic retinopathy
* Cotton wool spots – poorly defined bright patches (yellow/grey) due to infarction of the nerve fibres in background diabetic retinopathy or hypertensive retinopathy.
* Haemorrhages:
  * Blot – dense red patches in front of the retina as seen in preproliferative diabetic retinopathy
  * Vitreous – large, very dense thick red patches in front of the retina as seen in retinal detachment and proliferative retinopathy
  * Flame – large, bright yellow erratic patches indicative of retinal vein occlusion
* Drusen – bright yellow exudates behind the retina (as opposed to hard exudates, which are in front of the retina); age-related macular degeneration
* Panretinal laser photocoagulation scars – multiple pale yellow patches in the periphery of the retina
* Bone spicule pigmentation – retinitis pigmentosa.

Finishing off

* Thank the patient
* Make sure patient is comfortable and offer to help cover them up
* Wash hands
* Present and consider age of patient in forming differential
* Summarise.

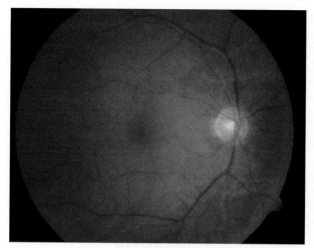

The normal fundus

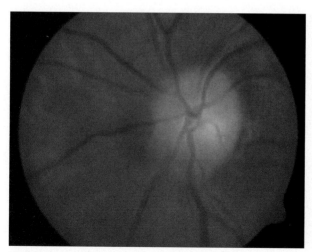

Blurred disk margin

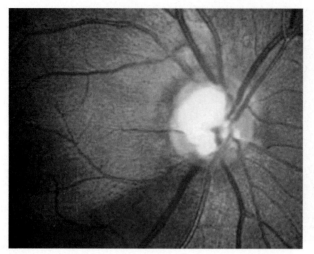

Increased cup:disk ratio

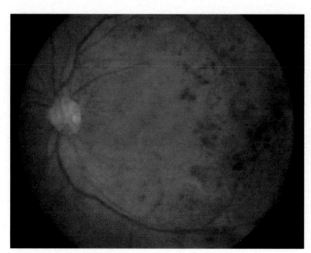

Neovascularisation in the disk: blot haemorrhages

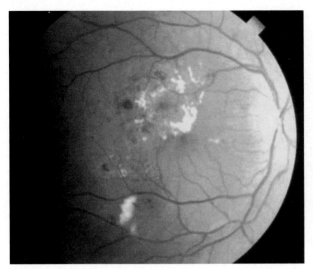

Micro-aneurysms, blot haemorrhages and hard exudates

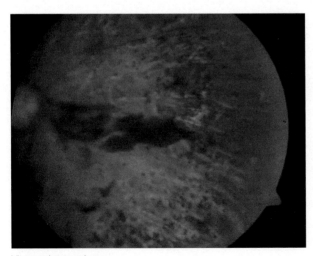

Vitreous haemorrhage

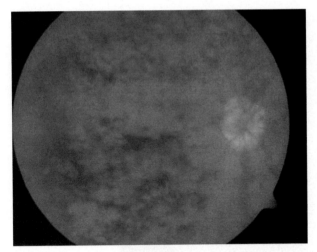

Flame haemorrhage

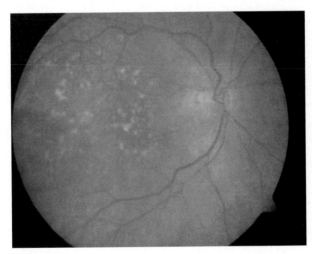

Drusen

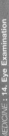

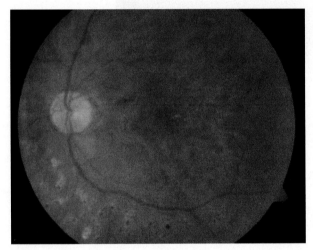

Laser scarring

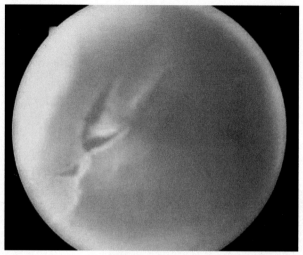

Retinal folds and retinal hole

Investigations

Nystagmus

Initial investigations are those of a cerebellar syndrome:

- MRI of brain, visual evoked potentials and CSF analysis for oilgoclonal bands to exclude multiple sclerosis
- MRI of brain to exclude posterior fossa tumours
- CT of brain to exclude stroke
- Thyroid function tests.

Ptosis and Horner's syndrome

- CT of brain (stroke)
- MRI of brain (demeyelination)
- Chest X-ray to exclude Pancoast's tumour.

IIIrd nerve palsy

- CT of brain
- Urine dipstick for glucose
- Thyroid function tests
- ESR in older patients to exclude temporal arteritis.

VIth nerve palsy

- CT of brain (VIth nerve palsy is a false localising sign in raised intracranial pressure)
- Urine dipstick for glucose
- Consider MRI of brain and CSF analysis in younger patients to exclude multiple sclerosis.

Homonymous hemianopia

- Formal visual field testing (perimetry)
- CT of brain (stroke, tumour).

Bitemporal hemianopia

- Formal visual field testing (perimetry)
- MRI of brain (pituitary adenoma)
- Serum prolactin (prolactinoma), glucose tolerance test (acromegaly).

Diabetic retinopathy

- HbA1c (an indicator of glycaemic control)
- Serum lipids
- U&E (renal function).

Thyroid Examination

1

Summary

☐ Patient seated with neck exposed

☐ Pulse

☐ Palms

☐ Tremor

☐ Eyes

☐ Thyroid palpation

☐ Thyroid auscultation

☐ Reflexes

Examiner's instruction

"Examine this patient's thyroid status and present your findings."

"This patient has noticed a swelling in her neck. Please examine it."

Wh Wash hands

I   Introduce yourself and identify patient (is the voice hoarse? – goitre)

S   Summarise that you would like to examine their thyroid function

P   Permission

E   Expose neck to the clavicles; equipment – sheet of paper, cup of water, tendon hammer

R   Reposition sitting up

S   State of patient (well/unwell); clues of current treatment

General inspection

Stand at the end of the bed and look at the patient

- Clothing (? Consistent with temperature)
- Weight status (thin/overweight)
- Behaviour (irritable/lethargic)
- Obvious tremor
- Skin changes (coarse and dry in hypothyroid states).

ACE TIPS

Ask the patient if they are in any pain before you touch them

---

Hands

Inspect

- Tremor (fine)
  - Ask patient to hold hands out, palms facing downwards
  - Lay a sheet of paper on the back of hands
- Other autoimmune disorders (e.g., vitiligo).
- Thyroid acropachy (pseudo-clubbing)
- Onycholysis
- Palmar erythema (thyrotoxicosis)
- BM stick marks (diabetes mellitus)
- Hyper-pigmented palmar creases (Addison's disease).

Palpation

- Warmth (shake hands with the patient)
- Sweaty palms
- Radial pulse – rate and rhythm
  - Bradycardia – consider hypothyroid states
  - Atrial fibrillation (AF) – consider hyperthyroid states.

Face

- "Peaches and cream complexion" (hypothyroid)
- Hair thinning
- Loss of lateral part of eyebrows.

Eyes

Inspect

- Pallor under eyelid
- Exophthalmos
- Lid retraction – visible white sclera above the iris
- Lid lag – ask patient to follow finger down with their eyes, keeping their head still. Look for a delay in eyelid shutting as the patient follows finger down.
- Ophthalmoplegia – ask patient to follow finger in H shape. Look for asymmetry of eye movement. Ask about double vision at each point.
- Periorbital oedema
- Chemosis and conjunctivitis.

Definitions of eye signs

Chemosis: swelling and ulceration of the conjunctiva.

Proptosis/exophthalmos: protrusion of the eye out of the orbit best seen from standing behind the patient.

Lid lag: slow movement or lagging of the upper eyelid on looking down.

Lid retraction: the sclera can be seen between.

ACE TIP

Proptosis, chemosis, ophthalmoplegia, acropachy and pretibial myxoedema are signs only seen in Graves' disease. Other signs occur in hyperthyroid states from any cause.

Werner's mnemonic for the progression of eye signs in Grave's disease (NO SPECS)

No signs or symptoms

Only lid retraction +/- lid lag

Soft tissue involvement

Proptosis

Extraocular muscle involvement

Corneal involvement

Sight loss due to optic nerve

From the front

Neck

Inspect

- Scars (collar scar from thyroid surgery)
- Asymmetry
- Deformity or visible lump
- Specific signs – goitre or thyroglossal cyst.

Special manoeuvres

- **Goitre:** ask patient to sip water and hold it in their mouth until you ask them to swallow. Feel for upward movement of a midline swelling on swallowing. Ask them to repeat this and feel inferiorly to the thyroid to assess retrosternal extension.
- **Thyroglossal cyst:** ask patient to stick tongue out. Feel for upward movement of a midline swelling.

Palpation

- Carotid pulse – character
- Tracheal position.

Auscultation

- Ask patient to briefly hold their breath.
- Using the diaphragm of the stethoscope, listen over the thyroid for bruit.

ACE TIP

The presence of a thyroid bruit is a very sensitive clinical sign of thyrotoxicosis.

> **Quick guide to assess thyroid status**
>
> - Pulse
> - Palms
> - Tremor
> - Eyes
> - Thyroid (including bruit)
> - Reflexes

From the back

Eyes

Inspect
- Exophthalmos – look over the top of patient's head for protruding eyes.

Neck

Palpation

Inform patient that you will feel their neck from behind and that it may be a little uncomfortable.
- Thyroid gland – standing behind the patient, use both hands for palpation. Fix one side of the thyroid with one hand and palpate with the other hand. If thyroid is enlarged: diffuse/localized. Describe characteristics of a lump: size, shape, texture (smooth/nodular), tender or non-tender.
- Anterior and posterior triangle lumps.
- Cervical lymphadenopathy.

Percussion
- Percuss down the upper part of the sternum. Dullness indicates retrosternal goitre.

Finishing off
- Thank the patient
- Make sure patient is comfortable and offer to help cover them up
- Wash hands
- Present and consider age of patient in forming differential
- Summarise.

Mention that you would:
- Inspect shins for pretibial myxoedema – this has an orange-peel texture (hypothyroidism).
- Check for difficulty in rising from sitting position (proximal myopathy).
- Check for slow relaxing reflexes.
- Ask the patient about symptoms of thyrotoxicosis.

Case presentation

"On examination, this lady has a large, multinodular goitre and a scar from a previous thyroidectomy. She has some signs of thyrotoxicosis, namely a tremor on examination, but she is not tachycardic at rest and the pulse is regular. She has no evidence of thyroid eye disease and I therefore conclude that she has thyrotoxicosis, secondary to a multinodular goitre."

"On examination, this lady has obvious signs of Graves' disease, namely exophthalmos, lid retraction and a thyroidectomy scar. She is clinically euthyroid at present as her pulse is normal at 72 beats per minute, regular rhythm. She does have a fine tremor, but no other signs of thyrotoxicosis at present. I would like to ask this patient about symptoms of thyrotoxicosis."

Investigations

- Thyroid function tests (TSH, T4 +/– T3)

- Thyroid autoantibodies

- A radio-iodine (^{131}I) scan shows increased uptake in Graves' disease and decreased uptake in thyroiditis

- Full blood count may show macrocytosis in hypothyroidism.

Cushing's Syndrome Examination

Examiner's instructions

"This patient has a long history of steroid use. Examine this patient as appropriate."

"The asthmatic man complains of weakness in his arms and legs. Please examine him and establish the cause"

> ### Cushing's disease and syndrome
>
> A constellation of signs and symptoms caused by persistently elevated glucocorticoid levels.
>
> • Cushing's disease results from elevated glucocorticoids due to excess production of ACTH from a pituitary adenoma.
>
> • Cushing's syndrome is elevated glucocorticoids from any cause.

Wh Wash hands

I Introduce yourself and identify patient

S Summarise that you would like to examine them

P Permission – listen for husky and deep voice

E Expose neck to the clavicles, and later the abdomen

R Reposition sitting up

S State of patient – look around bed for clues as to cause of Cushing's syndrome.

> ### Clues to the cause of Cushing's syndrome on inspection
>
> • Inhalers, nebulisers, oxygen – steroids used in COPD/ asthma/ fibrosing alveolitis
>
> • Colostomy/ ileostomy bag – inflammatory bowel disease
>
> • Transplant scars
>
> • Rheumatoid arthritis

General inspection

Stand at the end of the bed and look at the patient

Consequences of excess glucocorticoid

• Centripetal adiposity

• Moon-like facies

• Buffalo hump

• Hirsute – caused by exogenous steroids as they suppress adrenal androgen secretion

• Osteoporosis effects such as kyphosis.

Hands

Inspect

- Thin skin
- Bruising
- BM stick marks in diabetes
- Thin skin
- Bruising
- Pigmentation (ACTH)
- Poor wound healing
- Insulin injection sites.

> **ACE TIPS**
>
> Ask the patient if they are in any pain before you touch them

> **Causes of Cushing's syndrome**
>
> **Iatrogenic:** (therapeutic corticosteroids)
>
> **Cushing's disease:** pituitary adenoma causing excess ACTH resulting in excess cortisol secretion from the adrenals
>
> **Adrenocortical adenoma/carcinoma**
>
> **Ectopic ACTH secretion:** small cell carcinoma of the lung

Face

Inspect

- Moon-like facies
- Hirsute
- Acne
- Telangiectasia
- Look into mouth for oral thrush.

Special manoeuvre

- Check visual fields for field loss (pituitary adenoma, e.g., bitemporal hemianopia)

Neck

Inspect

- Look closely at interscapular area for "buffalo hump" as well as fat pads and bulge above supraclavicular fossae.

Chest and abdomen

Inspect

- Look for classical purple striae and skin thinning (can also be seen over shoulders and thighs).

Limbs

Inspect

• Look for bruising, muscle wasting and weakness of muscles of shoulders and hips.

• Assess for proximal myopathy (ask patient to rise from sitting in a chair with arms folded and test shoulder abduction).

• Look at lower limbs for evidence of peripheral oedema.

From the back

Inspect

• Look for evidence of osteoporosis and vertebral collapse e.g. kyphoscoliosis.

Finishing off

• Thank the patient

• Make sure patient is comfortable and offer to help cover them up

• Wash hands

• Present and consider age of patient in forming differential

• Summarise.

Mention that you would:

• Measure blood pressure

• Dipstick urine for glucose

• Assess visual fields if not already done

• Consider doing fundoscopy to seek hypertensive or diabetic retinopathy.

Case presentation

"This patient has a typical cushingoid appearance. I note that she is breathless at rest and the presence of inhalers at her bedside. This suggests that she is asthmatic and that she has iatrogenic Cushing's syndrome. There are abdominal needle marks, consistent with administration of insulin, implying that she has developed diabetes mellitus.

Investigations

Is the cortisol elevated?

• Urine – 24-hour urinary free cortisol: the most reliable test for cortisol secretion.

• Blood test:

  • Overnight or low-dose dexamethasone suppression test – if cortisol is suppressed in low-dose test: pseudo-Cushing's syndrome

  • Do high-dose dexamethasone suppression test – if cortisol is suppressed, the likely diagnosis is Cushing's disease

  • If cortisol is not suppressed in high-dose dexamethasone test, test serum ACTH levels.

What is the source?

- Serum ACTH:
  - Elevated if there is an (ectopic) ACTH secreting tumour (pituitary adenoma in Cushing's disease or small cell lung carcinoma)
  - Suppressed in cases of cortisol secreting adrenal adenoma or carcinoma.
- Imaging (directed by blood tests):
  - MRI of brain looking for pituitary microadenoma in Cushing's disease
  - Petrosal vein sampling
  - Chest X-ray looking for small cell lung cancers
  - Ultrasound scan looking for adrenal adenomas and carcinomas.

● Acromegaly Examination

Examiner's instructions

"This patient is suspected to have acromegaly. Examine this patient as appropriate."

"This lady has noticed that her shoes don't fit, Please examine her."

"Examine this patient who is sweating and has headaches."

> ### Acromegaly
>
> Acromegaly is a disorder of adults caused by hypersecretion of growth hormone by a benign pituitary adenoma. It is a diagnosis that can frequently be made on inspection. It is a common case in medical finals.

Wh Wash hands

I Introduce yourself and identify patient – while shaking hands note doughy texture of large spade-like hands

S Summarise that you would like to examine them

P Permission – listen for husky and deep voice

E Expose neck and chest

R Reposition sitting up

S State of patient

Signs around bed – old photographs (compare with present appearance).

General inspection

Stand at the end of the bed and look at the patient

- Increased foot and hand size (hands may be deliberately hidden, e.g., in pockets, under handbag)
- Increased head/hat size
- Excessive sweating
- Mildly hirsute
- Look briefly for signs of osteoarthritis (OA) such as kyphosis.

> ### ACE TIPS
>
> Ask the patient if they are in any pain before you touch them

Hands

Inspect

- Large
- Doughy
- Spade-shaped
- Signs of carpal tunnel syndrome (loss of thenar eminence with impaired sensation in median nerve distribution)

- Look at joints briefly for OA
- BM stick marks in diabetes.

Palpation

- Warmth
- Sweaty palms
- Hand enveloped in large doughy palm.

Face

Inspect

- Greasy skin with acne
- Large mandible
- Malocclusion of teeth (prognathism)
- Wide spaces between teeth
- Ask patient to stick tongue out (large with impressions of teeth on edges)
- Enlarged nose and ears
- Look for hypophysectomy scar under upper lip.

Eyes

Inspect

- Prominent supra-orbital ridges
- Examine visual fields to elicit bitemporal hemianopia.

Skin

Inspect

- Thick
- Multiple skin tags (associated with colonic polyps)
- Look in axillae for skin tags and acanthosis nigricans.

From the front

Examine for proximal myopathy:

- Ask patient to fold arms and stand from sitting
- Assess gait – rolling gait with bowed legs.

Listen to chest, assess JVP and look for pulmonary oedema in cardiac failure.

Finishing off

- Thank the patient
- Make sure patient is comfortable and offer to help cover them up
- Whash hands
- Present and consider age of patient in forming differential
- Summarise.

Mention that you would

- Measure blood pressure
- Fundoscopy to assess hypertensive or diabetic retinopathy
- Test the urine for glucose
- Recommend screening colonoscopy to look for polyps and colorectal cancers
- Chest X-ray and electrocardiogram (ECG) – cardiomegaly.

Case presentation

"This patient has acromegaly as evidenced by spade-like hands, loss of thenar eminence consistent with carpal tunnel syndrome. She has prominent supra-orbital ridges, with an enlarged jaw and prognathism. There is no evidence of a bitemporal hemianopia. I would like to dipstick the urine for glucose to check for diabetes mellitus, request a chest radiograph to assess possible cardiomegaly and perform an electrocardiogram."

Investigations:

- Blood tests – oral glucose tolerance test (for diagnosis)
- Plasma IGF-1 (usually for monitoring response to treatment)
- Imaging – MRI of brain (looking for pituitary adenoma). The majority of patients with acromegaly have a macroadenoma, which can be seen on MRI.
- Formal visual field testing
- ECG.

Summary

- ☐ Patient seated, both hands exposed and resting on a pillow or table top.

- ☐ Inspect for scars, asymmetry and deformities.

- ☐ Inspect nails for clubbing, pitting and onycholysis.

- ☐ Inspect the proximal interphalangeal joints (PIPJ) for Bouchard's nodes and gouty tophi.

- ☐ Inspect the distal interphalangeal joints (DIPJ) for Heberden's nodes.

- ☐ Look at the elbows for nodules.

- ☐ Turn the hands over and inspect the palmar surfaces for: scars, symmetry, muscle wasting at thenar and hypothenar eminences, Dupuytren's contracture, palmar erythema.

- ☐ Palpate across the wrist and metacarpophalangeal joint (MCPJ) lines feeling for warmth, swelling and tenderness.

- ☐ Palpate each of the MCPJ, PIPJ and DIPJ in turn.

- ☐ Actively move (flexion and extension) the wrist.

- ☐ Ask patient to bend and straighten the fingers and thumb.

- ☐ Assess motor and sensory function of the median and ulnar nerves of each hand.

- ☐ Perform Tinel's and Phalen's test to assess for the presence of carpal tunnel syndrome.

- ☐ Assess function, e.g., by asking the patient to pick up and pretend to sign their name, use a key, undo buttons on their shirt.

Examiner's instruction

"Examine this patient's hands and present your clinical findings."

Common OSCE cases

- Rheumatoid hands
- Osteoarthritis
- Psoriatic arthropathy
- Ulnar nerve palsy
- Radial nerve palsy
- Median nerve palsy
- Carpal tunnel syndrome
- Finger clubbing
- Scleroderma

Key signs for common OSCE cases

- **Rheumatoid arthritis:** symmetrical arthropathy principally affecting carpal, MCP and PIP joints. Ulnar deviation, Boutonniere deformity, swan-neck deformity, Z thumb +/– rheumatoid nodules. Generalised muscle wasting and palmar erythema.

- **Osteoarthritis:** asymmetrical arthropathy affecting the DIP (with Heberden's nodes) +/– PIP (with Bouchard's nodes).

- **Psoriatic arthropathy:** usually symmetrical arthropathy as for rheumatoid arthritis, but with nail changes and psoriatic skin plaques, particularly affecting the elbows and in the hair line.

- **Ulnar nerve palsy:** clawing of the fourth and fifth fingers. Sensory loss over medial one and half fingers.

- **Radial nerve palsy:** weakness of wrist and elbow extension. Fingers cannot be straightened.

- **Median nerve palsy/ carpal tunnel syndrome:** thenar eminence wasting, weakness of flexion, abduction and opposition of the thumb, reduced sensation over lateral three and a half fingers.

- **Clubbing:** an obvious appearance. Look for cyanosis, tar staining of the fingers and stigmata of thyroid disease.

- Add **scleroderma:** look for signs of systemic sclerosis including at the face for a beaked like nose and microstomia (reduced mouth opening). The hands will have telangiectasia, tight shiny skin (sclerodactyly), digital ischaemia and atrophy with subcutaneous calcinosis.

- Look for **Raynaud's phenomenon** and ask about oesophageal dysmotility indicating CREST syndrome.

Wh Wash hands

I Introduce yourself and identify patient

S Summarise how you would like to examine their hands

P Permission

E Expose both hands and wrists rolling sleeves above elbows

R Reposition patient – hands on lap, table or pillow palms up

S State of patient (well/unwell).

> **ACE TIPS**
>
> Ask the patient if they are in any pain before you touch them

Inspect

Dorsum

- Scars
- Asymmetry
  - Muscle wasting – hand intrinsics
  - Dactylitis
  - Swellings
- Deformity
  - Swan neck
  - Boutonnière's
  - Z thumb
  - Ulnar deviation of the fingers
- Specific
  - Nails – Clubbing, pitting, onycholysis
  - Wrist – synovitis
  - PIPJ – Bouchard's nodes, gouty tophi, Boutonnière's deformity
  - DIPJ – Heberden's nodes, psoriatic arthropathy, swan neck deformity
  - Elbow – rheumatoid nodules or psoriatic plaques.

Palmar

- Scars
- Asymmetry – muscle wasting: thenar/ hypothenar eminence
- Deformity – Dupuytren's contracture
- Specific – palmar erythema.

> **Palmar erythema**
>
> **Definition:** reddening of the palms of the hands, affecting the thenar and hypothenar eminences, and the soles of the feet
>
> **Causes:** liver disease, thyrotoxicosis, rheumatoid arthritis, pregnancy

> **Dupuytren's contracture**
>
> **Definition:** a fixed flexion contracture of the hand where the fingers bend towards the palm and cannot be fully extended
>
> **Causes:** family history, diabetes, liver disease, alcoholism, epilepsy and pulmonary, occupational trauma

Palpate

Describe any lumps found.

Dorsum

- Warmth across wrist and MCPJ lines
- Swelling and tenderness.

Wrist

- MCPJ – gently squeeze across the joint line of all MCP joints
- PIPJ – isolate each joint and assess in turn
- DIPJ – isolate each joint and assess in turn.

Palmar

- Thenar and hypothenar muscle wasting
- Palmar thickening – Dupuytren's contracture
- Trigger finger nodule.

Move

Wrist

- Passive and active flexion/ extension of the wrist

Fingers

- Screen – ask patient to bend and straighten fingers and thumb.

Special manoeuvres

Assess median and ulnar nerve function (motor and sensory).

Motor median nerve

- Abductor pollicis brevis – ask patient to place their hand flat on table palm upwards and to try to push their thumb towards the ceiling against your resistance
- Opponens pollicis brevis – ask patient to touch the tip of the little finger with their thumb and to resist your attempts to pull them apart.

> **Muscles supplied by the median nerve ("LOAF")**
>
> **L**ateral two lumbricals
>
> **O**pponens pollicis brevis
>
> **A**bductor pollicis brevis
>
> **F**lexor pollicis brevis

Motor ulnar nerve
- Interossei – finger abduction and adduction
  - Ask patient to resist you squeezing fingers together.
  - Ask patient to grip a sheet of paper between their fingers and to resist your attempts to pull it away.

Muscles supplied by the ulnar nerve in the hand	
Interossei	(**D**orsal interossei **ab**duct) "DAB"
	(**P**almar interossei **ad**duct) "PAD"
Muscles which move the little finger.	

Motor radial nerve
- Test for weakness of wrist and elbow extension.

Sensory median nerve
- Thenar eminence.

Sensory ulnar nerve
- Hypothenar eminence.

Sensory radial nerve
- First dorsal web space.

Carpal tunnel syndrome (often associated with median nerve palsy)
- Tinel's test – tap over carpal tunnel to elicit tingling in median nerve distribution.
- Phalen's test – flex wrists held for at least 1 minute, reproducing symptoms of tingling/numbness in median nerve distribution.
- Assess median nerve function as above.

Function
- Ask patient to pick up a pen and/or pretend to sign their name and to pick up and use a key.

Causes of carpal tunnel syndrome
Pregnancy, rheumatoid arthritis, hypothyroidism, acromegaly, amyloidosis

Finishing off
- Thank the patient
- Make sure patient is comfortable and offer to help cover them up
- Wash hands

- Present and consider age of patient in forming differential
- Summarise.

Case presentation

"On examination of this patient's hands, there was a scar over the metacarpophalangeal joints of the left hand and a Z scar over all of the fingers of the right hand, consistent with tendon surgery. There was subluxation of the metacarpophalangeal joints and ulnar deviation of the phalanges. There were swan neck deformities of all the fingers and swelling of the metacarpophalangeal joints and bilateral Z-shaped thumb deformities. There was wasting of the dorsal interossei and the thenar and hypothenar eminencies bilaterally with bilateral weakness of the median and ulnar nerves. There is no evidence of active disease, as there were no tender or hot joints and no soft tissue swelling. Function was relatively well-preserved as evidenced by adequate precision grip of the pen and use of a key. Vascular status was normal. These appearances are consistent with a diagnosis of rheumatoid arthritis."

Investigations

- **Carpal tunnel syndrome:** nerve conduction studies, then establish the cause. Investigations according to clinical suspicion. hCG (pregnancy); thyroid function tests; glucose tolerance test (acromegaly)
- **Ulnar nerve palsy:** nerve conduction studies
- **Radial nerve palsy:** nerve conduction studies
- **Generalised wasting of the hand muscles:** chest X-ray to exclude Pancoast's tumour.

Section II
Surgery

Examiner's instruction

"Examine this patient's lump and present your findings."

Common OSCE cases

- Lipoma
- Ganglion
- Sebaceous cyst
- Neurofibroma
- Papilloma
- Dermoid cyst
- Pigmented naevus
- Malignant melanoma
- Lymph node
- Keloid scar

Signs associated with common OSCE cases

- **Lipoma:** hemispherical swelling, well-defined edge, very mobile. Soft consistency and may fluctuate. Not attached to overlying skin. May be found anywhere in the body.

- **Ganglion:** hemispherical swelling, smooth surface, firm consistency commonly found near a joint or tendon. It may be weakly transluminable.

- **Sebaceous cyst:** hemispherical swelling, smooth surface, firm consistency. Attached to overlying skin and a central punctum may be present.

- **Neurofibroma:** soft, pedunculated swellings. Often multiple. As they arise from cutaneous nerves, they are mobile in transverse plane, but fixed in longitudinal plane. Look for café-au-lait spots suggesting neurofibromatosis.

- **Papilloma:** soft, pedunculated skin tag. May be found anywhere on the skin.

- **Dermoid cyst:** soft, spherical swelling. Smooth consistency, may fluctuate. Not attached to overlying skin or structures below. Classic sites of congenital dermoid cysts are medial or lateral to eyebrow (angular dermoids), but may occur at any site of fusion of skin dermatomes.

- **Pigmented naevus:** flat or raised pigmented lesion, with smooth edges and regular in colour. Halo naevus is a specific type with surrounding depigmentation. Hairy naevus is a congenital naevus, which may be very large with hair growth within.

Signs associated with common OSCE cases—cont'd

- **Malignant melanoma:** typically very darkly pigmented lesion, with irregularity in colour, irregular edges, may have ulceration. In practice unusual in examinations, as rapidly excised on diagnosis. More common would be recurrent melanomas.

- **Lymph node:** subcutaneous swelling of any size within lymphatic basins e.g., Cervical, axillary, inguinal, femoral. Characteristics depend on aetiology – a malignant lymph node is typically of hard consistency and immobile.

- **Keloid scar:** raised, red and often itchy scar.

Wh Wash hands

I Introduce yourself and identify patient

S Summarise how you would like to examine their lump

P Permission

E Expose the relevant area keeping the patient's dignity; equipment – measuring tape, pen torch, stethoscope

R Reposition to get the best view of the lump

S State of patient (well/unwell).

Do they have any other similar lumps?

ACE TIPS

Ask the patient if they are in any pain before you touch them

Inspect
- Site
- Size
- Shape
- Edge
- Colour
- Scars
- Skin changes (a punctum indicates a sebaceous cyst).

Be sure to look at the opposite limb for similar lumps.

Palpate
- Tender
- Warmth – use the back of the hands to compare warmth over the surface to the surroundings
- Surface – smooth/rough
- Consistency – hard, firm, rubbery, soft

- Edge
- Cough impulse
- Percuss – dull/resonant.

Move
Mobility
- The degree of mobility of a lump can be used to determine where the lump originates.

Origin
- Skin:
  - Pinch the skin
  - Asses whether lump rises with it
- Subcutaneous layer:
  - Pinch the skin with right hand
  - Move lump with left hand in a cross sign movement
  - Asses if lump moves independent of skin above
- Muscle:
  - Tense the underlying muscle group
  - Asses if lump moves
  - If lump does not move, it originates from or is fixed to muscle

Pulsatile (e.g., aneurysm)
- Lay a finger from each hand on either side of the lump
- Fingers pushed upwards – transmitted pulsation
- Fingers pushed outwards – expansile pulsation.

Fluid tests:
- Fluctuance – for small lumps (e.g., sebaceous cyst):
  - Lay two fingers from the same hand on either end of the lump.
  - Compress the lump with a finger from the opposite hand.
  - Look to see if the two fingers move apart, indicative of fluctuance
- Fluid thrill – for big lumps (e.g., ascites)
  - Patient rests the side of their hand in the centre of the lump
  - Flick the lump at one end
  - Feel for a transmission impulse at the other end.

Transillumination
- Using a pen torch shine a light behind the swelling
- Assess intensity of illumination on the front of the swelling.

Reducibility (e.g., haemangioma)
- Gently apply pressure to the swelling
- Assess whether swelling disappears

• Keeping hand in same position, ask the patient to cough
• Feel for a cough impulse.

Auscultate

• Bruit
• Machinery murmur of arteriovenous malformation
• Bowel sound.

Finishing off

• Thank the patient
• Make sure patient is comfortable and offer to help cover them up
• Wash hands
• Present and consider age of patient in forming differential
• Summarise.

Mention that you would like to

• Palpate lymph nodes
• Examine neurovascular status of area
• Observe for similar lumps in other areas.

Case presentation

"In summary, this gentleman has a 3 cm by 3 cm lump over the lateral malleolus of the right ankle. It is fluctuant and transluminable. These findings are consistent with a ganglion."

Investigations

• Many of these lesions can be confidently diagnosed clinically, and may not require any further investigation.
• Ultrasound may differentiate solid from cystic lesions.
• Pigmented lesions may require dermatoscopy or biopsy (excision biopsy if small, incision biopsy if large).

◉ Ulcer Examination

Examiner's instruction

"Examine this patient's lesion and present your findings."

Common OSCE cases

- Venous ulcer
- Arterial ulcer
- Neuropathic ulcer
- Mixed ulcers
- Basal cell carcinoma
- Squamous cell carcinoma

Signs associated with common OSCE cases

- **Venous ulcer:** typically in "gaiter" area over medial calf. Look for haemosiderin deposition, lipodermatosclerosis (thin tight shiny skin) and visible varicose veins or previous scars from varicose vein surgery.

- **Arterial ulcer:** painful punched out ulcer (vertical edges), necrosis (black) with absent pulses.

- **Neuropathic ulcer:** painless ulcer within pressure area (e.g., sole of foot) with reduced sensation. Typically in diabetics.

- **Mixed ulcers:** mixed features.

- **Basal cell carcinoma:** classic pearly white appearance with rolled edges and telangiectasia.

- **Squamous cell carcinoma:** raised keratotic lesion with everted edges. May have regional lymphadenopathy.

Wh Wash hands

I Introduce yourself and identify patient

S Summarise how you would like to examine their ulcer

P Permission – ask about removing any dressing in any examination

E Expose the relevant area preserving the patient's dignity; equipment – measuring tape

R Reposition to get the best view of the ulcer

S State of patient (well/unwell), nicotine stained, short of breath, obese, cachectic, varicose veins

Signs around bed – walking aid, insulin, cigarettes or lighter

"Do you have anything else similar on your body?"

> **ACE TIPS**
>
> Ask the patient if they are in any pain before you touch them

Basics
- Site
- Size
- Shape.

Base
- Colour – red (healthy granulation tissue), pale pink (ischaemia), white (slough), black (necrotic tissue)
- State visible anatomical structures – tendons or bones indicates arterial cause.

Depth
- Estimate height (mm).

> **Arterial ulcers**
>
> Painful; affect the distal extremities and pressure points; associated with absent pulses and thin, hairless skin.

Edge
- Flat sloping edge – typically venous
- Punched-out edge – typically arterial or neuropathic
- Undermined ulcer – typically pressure sores
- Rolled edge – typical of basal cell carcinoma
- Everted edge – typical of a squamous carcinoma.

> **Neuropathic ulcers**
>
> Painless; affect pressure areas; associated with peripheral neuropathy.

Discharge
- Serous – clear
- Sanguineous – blood
- Purulent – pus.

> **Venous ulcers**
>
> Painless; affect the gaiter area of the leg; associated with venous hypertension (varicose veins, oedema, atrophie blanche).

Surroundings

- Colour
- Scars
- Skin changes:
  - Venous – lipodermatosclerosis, haemosiderosis.
  - Arterial – loss of hair, dusky skin colour, cool skin.

ACE TIPS

Look for the cause:

- Venous – pelvic mass
- Arterial – pale, cold, pulseless limbs
- Neuropathic – evidence of diabetes mellitus

Finishing off

- Thank the patient
- Make sure patient is comfortable and offer to help cover them up
- Wash hands
- Present and consider age of patient in forming differential
- Summarise.

Mention that you would like to

- Neurovasculature – assess sensation and feel pulses
- Lymph nodes – enlargement, tenderness
- Assess previously healed ulcers.

Case presentation

"In summary, this gentleman is a known diabetic with a 1 cm by 1 cm lesion on the anterior aspect of the left lower limb. There is loss of hair and a shiny, thin skin appearance with a surrounding area of erythema, which could be healed granulation tissue or haemosiderin deposition associated with venous disease. This has the appearance of a healed diabetic ulcer."

◉ Neck Examination

The examination of the neck is often confused with that of the thyroid system, as the patients in this OSCE station commonly have thyroid goitres. If the instruction states that you should examine the neck, and a goitre is found, you should complete the examination as described below, and only then should you proceed to assess the thyroid system (see thyroid chapter), explaining your reasoning to the examiner.

Examiner's instruction

"This gentleman has found a lump in his neck. Please examine his neck."

Common OSCE cases

Any of the common lesions listed under lumps and bumps may occur in the neck.

- Lymphadenopathy
- Branchial cyst
- Thyroid nodules
- Thyroglossal cyst
- Pharyngeal pouch
- Cystic hygroma
- Chemodectoma/carotid body tumour

Signs associated with common OSCE cases

Anterior triangle:

- Lymphadenopathy (firm/rubbery)

- Branchial cyst (smooth, firm, fluctuates transilluminates)

- Chemodectoma (firm and pulsatile, related to carotid artery)

Posterior triangle:

- Lymphadenopathy

- Pharyngeal pouch (cystic swelling, patient has halitosis and may regurgitate undigested food)

- Cystic hygroma (child with a soft, fluctuant swelling which transilluminates brilliantly)

Midline:

- Thyroid nodules (moves upwards with swallowing)

- Thyroglossal cyst (moves upwards with tongue protrusion)

Wh Wash hands

I Introduce yourself and identify patient

S Summarise what you would like to examine

P Permission

E Expose the chest down to the waist

R Reposition on a chair

S State of patient – well/unwell, old/young

Signs around bed – glass of water may indicate a thyroid lump, tablets (carbimazole or thyroxine).

ACE TIPS

• Ask patient if they are in any pain or noticed any lumps before you touch them.

• Make sure patient is sitting on a chair away from wall.

Inspect

• Obvious goitre or other neck lumps
• Describe the characteristics of any swelling:
    • Site – describe in terms of the triangles of the neck/ midline
    • Size
    • Shape
    • Colour

Definitions

Anterior triangle: anterior border of sternocleidomastoid, midline and ramus of mandible

Posterior triangle: posterior border of sternocleidomastoid, anterior border of trapezius and clavicle

---

• Scars – thyroidectomy (collar incision), carotid endarterectomy (anterior border of sternocleidomastoid)
• Ask the patient to swallow (give the patient a glass of water)
    • Inspect whether the swelling moves upwards with swallowing – likely to be related to thyroid
• Ask patient to protrude the tongue
    • A thyroglossal cyst will move upwards due to its attachment to foramen caecum at base of tongue.

Palpate from behind
- Start by feeling the lump itself and describe its characteristics:
  - Tender
  - Warmth – use the back of the hands to compare warmth over the surface to the surroundings
  - Size
  - Shape
  - Edge
  - Surface – smooth/rough
  - Consistency – hard, firm, rubbery, soft
  - Mobility
  - Pulsatile
  - Transillumination (if appropriate)

> **ACE TIPS**
>
> If the lesion is arising from the thyroid then palpate rest of thyroid for possible multinodular goitre.

- Repeat the actions of swallowing and tongue protrusion to confirm the lump moves with these actions
- Move onto examining the groups of lymph nodes:
  - Submental
  - Submandibular
  - Anterior cervical
  - Posterior cervical
  - Supraclavicular
  - Pre-auricular
  - Post-auricular
  - Occipital
- Palpate the muscles (sternocleidomastoids and trapezius)
- Feel the carotid pulses (Do not feel both pulses at the same time)

Auscultation
- Carotid bruits
- Thyroid bruits

Finishing off
Perform a complete examination of the thyroid system if the lesion is arising from thyroid gland.
- Thank the patient
- Make sure patient is comfortable and offer to help cover them up
- Wash hands
- Present and consider age of patient in forming differential
- Summarise.

Mention that you would

- Examine the reticuloendothelial system if lymph nodes are enlarged

Investigations

- Many of these lumps have classical clinical appearances and can be confidently diagnosed clinically
- Ultrasound is the usual initial investigation
- Fine needle aspiration cytology may be performed on solid lumps
- Lymph nodes – blood tests to determine cause; full blood count and peripheral smear, liver function tests, ESR, glandular fever serology
- Barium swallow to diagnose pharyngeal pouch
- Carotid body tumour would require duplex ultrasound and angiography
- CT may be used to diagnose complex lumps.

💿 Breast Examination

Examiners instructions

"This patient is complaining of a lump in the breast. Please examine her."

Common OSCE cases

- Young lady with a fibroadenoma
- Breast cancer
- Previous breast cancer with or without recurrence
- Previous mastectomy with or without breast reconstruction
- Fibrocystic change
- Normal breasts
- Male with gynaecomastia

Key signs associated with common OSCE cases

- **Fibroadenoma:** a young patient with single or multiple well defined and extremely mobile breast lumps ("breast mouse"). Differential diagnosis is a cyst, which may be fluctuant or tender, and typically occurs in older patients. Ultrasound differentiates well.

- **Breast cancer:** a woman (or man) with an irregular, usually non-tender lump in the breast. May be fixed to skin (causing dimpling) or muscle. Can be bilateral!

- **Previous breast cancer:** a mastectomy or wide local excision scar. Signs of previous radiotherapy (skin tattoo or telangiectasia). Examine carefully around the scar for a clear lump and feel for lymph node metastases.

- **Previous mastectomy with or without breast reconstruction:** a mastectomy scar overlying a reconstructed breast. Look for a scar on the back or lower abdomen, as the donor site for reconstruction. Patient may have lymphoedema.

- **Fibrocystic change:** a young or perimenopausal patient with symmetrical often tender nodularity, most marked in upper outer quadrants.

- **Normal breasts:** may appear in the OSCE! If you have systematically examined the breasts and not found ANY abnormality, then say so!

- **Male with gynaecomastia:** young or old male patient with unilateral or bilateral breast lumps, which may be tender to touch. Ask them about medication they are taking.

Wh Wash hands

I Introduce yourself and identify patient

S Summarise that you would like to examine the patient's breasts

P Permission

E Expose the chest down to the waist

R Reposition sitting on the side of a bed for inspection. Palpation will be performed with the patient lying in bed at 45 degrees.

S State of patient (well/unwell)

Signs around bed.

ACE TIPS

- Ask the patient if they are in any pain or noticed any lumps before you touch them.

- Ensure you have a chaperone present and you have a private cubicle or side room.

Patient sitting

Inspect

Stand opposite the patient.

- Raise patients arms slowly above head (stretches Cooper's ligaments – suspensory ligaments of the breast), looking for:
  - Scars – previous mastectomy, lumpectomy, breast reduction
  - Radiotherapy tattoos
  - Asymmetry
  - Deformity
  - Skin changes
    - Puckering
    - Peau d'orange (orange peel skin)
  - Nipple
    - Retraction
    - Discharge
    - Destruction
    - Eczema (Paget's disease of the breast).
- Ask patient to place both hands on hips and to press down to tense the pectoralis major muscle, looking again for the above features.
- Lift up breast to look at the infra-mammary part of the breast.

Patient lying

Palpate

Start with the normal side.

- Feel with the flat of the hand systematically through the following areas:
  - 4 quadrants – feel in upper outer quadrant last, don't forget that it extends all the way into the axilla.
  - Centrally around the nipple (second most common location of a tumour in the breast)
  - Examine and describe the lump (as for any lump – see station on lumps):
    - Size
    - Mobility – free, tethered
  - Fixity to underlying muscle/overlying skin
    - Move lump in two directions
    - Repeat with patients hand pressed into hips
    - This determines attachment to pectoralis major.

Nipple

- Attempt to evert nipple if inverted (best to ask the patient to do this in an exam situation)
- It is usually considered better to ask the patient to express the discharge themselves if they can
- Massage areola from the areolar margin towards the nipple to assess presence and colour of discharge. Note whether the discharge is from a single duct or from multiple ducts. If a discharge is present, tell the examiner that you would test it for occult blood, using a urine dipstick.

Axilla

- Take the patient's right elbow with your right hand, supporting the weight of her arm. Examine for lympadenopathy in the 5 axillary areas:
  - Medial
  - Lateral

- Anterior
- Posterior
- Apical.
- Repeat for the opposite side.

Finishing off

- Thank the patient
- Comfort/ cover
- Wash hands
- Present and consider age of patient in forming differential
- Summarise.

Mention that you would

- Inspect the arms for signs of lymphoedema – compare left with right, and measure the arm circumference if in doubt
- Feel for cervical, supraclavicular and infraclavicular lymphadenopathy
- Examine the abdomen for hepatomegaly (metastases)
- Percuss for spinal tenderness (metastases)
- Perform triple assessment by imaging (with mammography or ultrasound or both) and biopsy (fine needle or core).
- Obtain a detailed history focusing on risk factors for breast cancer.

Investigations

The principle is that any breast lump should undergo "triple assessment", with all three aspects of triple investigation in agreement:

- Clinical evaluation (risk profiling, history and examination)
- Radiological evaluation (mammography and/or ultrasound). Young patients should initially be assessed by ultrasound as, in mammography, X-ray penetration is limited by dense breast tissue, and exposes breasts to radiation. MRI is a newer imaging modality that has excellent sensitivity
- Pathological evaluation (typically fine needle aspiration biopsy or core biopsy). If these fail to establish the diagnosis, then surgical biopsy (excision biopsy) may be required.

Examiner's instruction

"This patient is complaining of a lump in the groin. Please examine him/her."

Common OSCE cases

- Inguinal hernia (direct or indirect) – a large indirect inguinal hernia may extend into the scrotum, i.e., an inguinoscrotal hernia
- Femoral hernia
- Scrotal swelling
- Lymph node in the groin
- Saphenovarix
- Femoral aneurysm

Definition of a hernia

An abnormal protrusion of a viscus or organ through its containing cavity.

Groin anatomy basics

Successful diagnosis of groin lumps requires identification of the anatomical landmarks:

- Anterior superior iliac spine

- Pubic tubercle – which is the first bony prominence felt 45 degree inferomedial to the anterior superior ileac spine (ASIS)

- The inguinal ligament lies between the ASIS and the pubic tubercle

- The superficial inguinal ring lies superomedial to the pubic tubercle. All inguinal hernias reduce at this point. Femoral hernias reduce inferolateral to the pubic tubercle

- The deep inguinal ring lies at the *midpoint of the inguinal ligament*. The midpoint of the inguinal ligament is located half way between the anterior superior iliac spine and the pubic tubercle. Indirect hernias can be controlled by pressure over the deep inguinal ring

- Don't be confused by the *"mid-inguinal point"* – which lies midway between the pubic symphysis and the ASIS. This is where the femoral artery lies.

Signs associated with common OSCE cases

- **An inguinal hernia** (direct or indirect), if reducible, will reduce above and medial to the pubic tubercle (at the superficial inguinal ring). Inguinal hernias are the most common groin hernias (even in females). *Direct hernias* bulge directly through the superficial ring. *Indirect hernias* first pass through the deep ring, and then through the superficial ring. Clinical examination differentiates direct from indirect, though is not completely accurate, even when done by experienced surgeons.

- **Femoral hernias**, if reducible, will reduce below and lateral to the pubic tubercle (at the femoral canal) are more common in females than males (though inguinal hernia remains the most common groin hernia in females).

- **Differentiation of inguinoscrotal from scrotal swellings** is based on being able to get above the swelling in scrotal swellings.

- **Sapheno-varix** is very soft fluctuant swelling, similar in location to a femoral hernia, but typically in a patient with varicose veins.

- **Femoral aneurysm**: Expansile pulsatile swelling in the groin below the inguinal ligament. If you find a femoral aneurysm, look for an abdominal aortic and popliteal aneurysm.

Wh Wash hands

I Introduce yourself and identify patient

S Summarise what you would like to examine (groin)

P Permission

E Expose the patients – NO underwear – ensure adequate privacy and temperature

R Reposition the patient – standing

S State of patient (well/unwell)

Signs around bed – trusses.

ACE TIPS

Ask the patient if they are in any pain before you touch them

Standing

Inspect

- Swelling characteristics:
  - Site
  - Size
  - Colour e.g., overlying skin erythema
  - Scars (incisional hernia)
- Scrotum – does lump extend to scrotum?
- Ask the patient if they can reduce the lump.

Palpate

- Both sides – start on the normal side
- Swelling characteristics:

- Tender
- Warmth
- Consistency
- Reducible – attempt to reduce the lump yourself, if the patient has not already done so
- Cough impulse:
  - Attempt to reduce the swelling
  - Patient gives two big coughs (facing away)
  - Does swelling get bigger or more tense?
- If lump is in scrotum – can you get above it? This differentiates scrotal from inguinoscrotal swellings.

Auscultation

- Bowel sounds.

Femoral or inguinal

By now you will have identified that the swelling within the groin is a hernia. Proceed to identify whether the hernia is femoral or inguinal in origin.

Feel for landmarks

- Anterior superior iliac spine
- Pubic tubercle
- Superficial inguinal ring – just above and medial to pubic tubercle
- Deep inguinal ring – midpoint of the inguinal ligament (located midway between the pubic tubercle and the anterior superior iliac spine).

Reducibility

- If reduction is possible, note the position of reduction in relation to the pubic tubercle (this is the true site of a hernia).

Examination tip

- **An inguinal hernia** (direct or indirect), if reducible, will reduce above and medial to the pubic tubercle (at the superficial inguinal ring).

- **A femoral hernia**, if reducible, will reduce below and lateral to the pubic tubercle (at the femoral canal).

Direct or indirect

If you have identified an inguinal hernia, now identify whether it is direct or indirect.

Feel for landmarks

- Deep/internal inguinal ring (DIR) – midpoint of the inguinal ligament (located midway between the pubic tubercle and the anterior superior iliac spine)

Examination tip

- Indirect – controlled by pressure over **DIR**

- Direct – controlled by pressure over **SIR**

- After successful reduction, place pressure with a finger over the deep inguinal ring and ask the patient to cough. If the hernia is controlled then it is an indirect hernia. If not then it is more likely to be a direct hernia.

Finishing off

- Thank the patient
- Comfort/cover
- Wash hands
- Present and consider age of patient in forming differential
- Summarise.

Mention that you would:

- Examine external genitalia
- Perform a full abdominal examination.

Investigations

- Investigations are rarely required to diagnose groin hernias
- Ultrasound may, however, be used
- Scrotal swelling – ultrasound
- Lymph nodes may require ultrasound and fine needle aspiration biopsy. CT of the abdomen may be performed if lymphoma is suspected. Ultimately, lymph node biopsy may be required to diagnose the cause of the lymphadenopathy.
- Saphenovarix femoral aneurysm should be confirmed on duplex ultrasound. Angiography would be required to investigate an aneurysm further.

Testes or Scrotal Examination

Examiner's instruction

"Please examine this gentleman's scrotum."

Common OSCE cases:
- Hydrocoele
- Epididymal cyst
- Inguinoscrotal swelling (hernia)
- Patient with orchidectomy

Signs associated with common OSCE cases

- **Hydrocoele:** fluctuant swelling within which the testis cannot be felt; transilluminates.

- **Epididymal cyst:** fluctuant swelling felt adjacent to the testis; transilluminates.

- **Inguinoscrotal swelling (hernia):** cannot get above swelling.

- **Patient with orchidectomy:** single testicle felt within scrotum. Inguinal surgical scar which looks like a hernia repair.

Wh Wash hands

I Introduce yourself and identify patient

S Summarise that you would like to examine the testes

P Permission

E Expose fully the groin and external genitalia, using a blanket to cover and maintain dignity when not examining; equipment – measuring tape or beads, Put on a pair of gloves

R Reposition asking patient to lie on their back

S State of patient (well/unwell), abnormal masses visible from end of the bed.

Inspect
- Swellings
- Rash
- Ulcers
- Pubic hair distribution
- Scars
    - Inguinal
    - Midline scrotal scar suggests past expiration procedure of testis, e.g., after torsion.

- Asymmetry – check for symmetry in size and folds of scrotum
- Oedema of penis and scrotum (associated with congestive cardiac failure and nephrotic syndrome).

Remember to lift up the scrotum to inspect the ventral aspect.

If one testis is absent

Think:

- Cryptorchidism

- Surgical removal

- Retractile testicle – can be milked into the scrotum

Palpate

- Scrotum:
  - Palpate for any abnormal lumps in the scrotal skin – describe its characteristics as with any lump

ACE TIP

Ask the patient if they are in any pain or have noticed any lumps before you touch them

- Spermatic cord
  - Gently lifting the scrotal sac, palpate the spermatic cord tracing it from the inguinal ligament to the testes using thumb and index finger.
- Testes and epididymis

Characteristics of normal testes

- The left testis is lower than the right

- Testis is smooth, firm and rubbery

- Testis is 4–5 cm in length, 2.5 cm in breadth, 20–25 ml in volume and weighs 10.5–14 g

- There is a cord-like structure called the epididymis on each side adjacent to the testis

---

- The size of each testis should be measured with measuring beads
- Palpate the testes and epididymis, feeling for any abnormal swellings or tenderness. Describe the characteristics of the swelling as for any lump
- Assess transillumination of any swelling
- If you find any abnormal swellings, you must answer these two questions:
  - Is the lump separate from the testes?
  - Can you get above the lump?

Diagnosis

If you can get above it and the lump is not separate from the testis:

- **Hydrocoele** (fluid in the tunica vaginalis that transilluminates)

- **Haematocoele:** similar to hydrocoele but unlike hydrocoele, does not transilluminate. Usually accompanied with a history of trauma or following hydrocoele drainage

- **Tumour:** hard, non-tender, heavy and irregular testes that will need orchidectomy. Commonest malignancy in males aged 15–44 years

- **Orchitis:** large and tender testes. Unlikely in an exam unless it's a simulated patient

- **Testicular torsion:** unilateral, tender scrotal mass. Unlikely in an exam

Diagnosis

You can get above it and it is separate from the testis:

- **Epididymal cyst**

- **Epididymitis:** diffuse tenderness in epididymis

- **Varicocoele:** unilateral, non-tender mass adjacent to testis sometimes referred to as "a bag of worms" and most noticeable when standing. Not transilluminable

- **Hydrocoele of cord:** solitary transilluminable lump. Moves down with traction of testes

- **Spermatocoele:** small, non-tender nodule above and behind the Epididymal head containing clear or milky fluid. Typically occurs after vasectomy – so look for the scars. Typically vasectomy scars are found behind the scrotum where it connects to the perineum or on top of the scrotum (difficult to see)

Diagnosis

If you can not get above the lump, the lump is a hernia.

Finishing off
- Thank the patient
- Ask if they need any help getting dressed
- Wash hands
- Present findings
- Summarise.

Mention that you would:

- Examine the inguinal region for hernias and lymphadenopathy
- Carry out a full abdominal and respiratory examination looking for other abdominal masses and pleural effusions respectively.

Investigations

- Ultrasound
- Tumour markers – alpha-fetoprotein and beta-human chorionic gonadotropin (β-hCG).

Rectal Examination

It is almost unheard-of for rectal examination to appear in any OSCE, but it is such an important part of the abdominal exam that it warrants at least a few lines in this book.

There may be a dummy within the examination. The examiner will want to ensure that you get consent for the procedure, ensure a chaperone and treat the patient with dignity. You should perform the examination systematically, and invariably the pathology will be a palpable abnormal lump.

Make sure you ALWAYS mention that you would perform a rectal examination in the abdominal examination station, as well as in any urological stations (to assess prostate size).

Wh Wash hands

I Introduce yourself and identify patient

S Summarize that you would like to examine the patient's rectum

P Permission

E Expose the patient below the waist

R Reposition lying in the left lateral position

S State of patient (well/unwell)

Signs around bed.

ACE TIPS

- Obtain verbal consent from the patient and ensure presence of a chaperone.

- Ask the patient if they are in any pain or noticed any lumps before you touch them.

Patient lying

- Make sure patient is lying in the left lateral position Knees and hips flexed such that knees are as near to the chest as possible.
- Put on gloves and put lubricant jelly only your finger.

Inspect

- Are there any obvious lesions around the anus?
  - Describe the lesion in terms of size, shape, site, skin changes etc.
  - Ask the patient to bear down as you inspect – you may see prolapsing haemorrhoids or rectal mucosal prolapse
- Haemorrhoids – dilated anal cushions usually soft and compressible
  - If blue and tender – consider thrombosed haemorrhoids
  - May be internal or external, reducible or non-reducible
  - Describe site in terms of a clock imposed in the lithotomy position – the standard positions are at 3, 7 and 11 o'clock

- Anal fissures – tears along the anal canal, which appear white in colour
  - Very tender to touch, mainly in the posterior wall of anal canal
  - Patient is unlikely to be able to tolerate digital examination
- Perianal abscess – indurated area with surrounding cellulitis
  - Look for a midline pit to exclude pilonidal disease.
  - Also look for possible fistulation (e.g., constant discharge)

Digital palpation

- Using lubrication (e.g., KY jelly) insert the index finger of right hand. Ask the patient to relax, apply gentle pressure with the distal pulp of the finger, gently insert your finger
  - Palpate the posterior, anterior and both lateral walls in turn
- Feel for any obvious lesions and describe, as with any other lesions
  - Once again, describe the position according to the clock face
- Assess resting anal tone and squeeze pressure
  - E.g., extent of abscess, presence of internal haemorrhoids etc.
- On the anterior wall in a male, palpate the prostate
  - Describe its shape (bi-lobed, regular or irregular etc.)
  - Size and tenderness (e.g., prostatitis)
- Feel for any obvious hard stools within rectum or whether it is empty
- Finish by looking at the glove
  - Any blood or faeces (describe colour e.g., melaena).

Finishing off

- Give patient tissue paper to wipe themselves
- Thank the patient
- Ask if they need any help getting dressed
- Wash hands
- Present findings
- Summarise.

Mention that you would:

- Elicit a family history of bowel cancer and inflammatory bowel disease
- Perform a full abdominal examination (this includes looking in the mouth (for aphthous ulcers).

⊙ Peripheral Arterial Examination

Examiner question

"This gentleman is complaining of pain in his calf/thigh/buttocks on walking. Please examine the arterial system of the lower limbs."

"This patient has an ulcer over their lower leg/foot. Please examine the arterial system of the lower limbs."

Common OSCE cases

- Abdominal aortic aneurysm
- Peripheral aneurysm
- Peripheral vascular disease with missing pulses
- Abdominal scars
- Diabetic foot
- Bypass graft
- Patient who has undergone an amputation
- Arterial ulcers
- Renal dialysis patient with a surgical arteriovenous fistula
- Gangrene
- Raynaud's disease
- Acute arterial ischaemia needs urgent surgical treatment so these cases will not appear in examinations!

Signs associated with common OSCE cases

- **Abdominal aortic aneurysm:** expansile and pulsatile mass in the abdomen, to the left of the midline.

- **Peripheral aneurysm:** commonly popliteal or femoral. Think about this if you feel a popliteal pulse very easily!

- **Peripheral vascular disease with missing pulses:** nicotine stained patient, with chronic atrophic changes in the leg, with absent pulses in a cold limb. Levels involved may be aortoiliac, femoropopliteal or distal vessels.

- **Abdominal scars:**

  - Midline laparotomy for emergency AAA repair and any aortobifemoral bypass.

  - Transverse abdominal incision for an elective AAA repair.

- **Bypass graft:** aortobifemoral bypass graft will leave you with a laparotomy scar and vertical scars bilaterally over the inguinal ligament.

Signs associated with common OSCE cases—cont'd

- **Coronary artery bypass graft:** mid-sternotomy scar and long, vertical saphenous vein harvest scars on the legs.

- **Diabetic foot:** patient with a warm limb with ulceration or distal gangrene.

- **Patient who has undergone an amputation:** this may be above knee, below knee, trans-metatarsal or amputation of digits. If multiple amputations of digits in a young person – think of Buerger's disease.

- **Arterial ulcers:** similar features to peripheral vascular disease, but with ulceration. The classical appearance of an arterial ulcer is punched out.

- **Renal dialysis patient with a surgical arteriovenous fistula:** collapsing pulse, venous dilatation with a pulsation within, surgical scar on radial surface of forearm.

- **Gangrene:** may be due to diabetes or peripheral vascular disease.

- **Raynaud's disease:** female with pale or blue fingers and classic atrophy of nail pulp. Associated with collagen-vascular diseases such as scleroderma (which has a characteristic facies). Note that Raynaud's disease is distinct from Raynaud's phenomenon, which is simply change in colour from white to blue to crimson in response to cold exposure.

Wh Wash hands

I Introduce yourself and identify patient

S Summarise what you would like to examine

P Permission

E Expose the patients legs up to underwear

R Reposition patient supine (recline patient flat, head supported by pillow)

S State of patient (well/unwell)

Signs around bed – walking sticks, oxygen supply, drips/lines, pack of cigarettes

ACE TIP

Ask the patient if they are in any pain before you touch them

Arms

Inspect

- Nicotine staining
- Peripheral cyanosis
- Gangrene
- Arteriovenous fistula.

Palpate

- Temperature of both hands, forearms and arms
- Capillary refill time at finger nails

- Peripheral pulses on both sides:
  - Radial – with patients palm facing up, place two fingers lightly over the "groove" just palpable below the thumb
  - Brachial – use thumb or two fingers; pulse is located just medial to biceps tendon in antecubital fossa. Easier to palpate with the patient's arm in full extension at elbow
  - Grade pulses – absent, weak, normal, increased, bounding; if any are weak or diminished, then auscultate for bruits
  - Radioradial delay
- *The Allen test:*
  - Ask the patient to lift up their hand and make a fist
  - This position should be held for around 30 seconds
  - Occlude both the radial and ulnar arteries at wrist by applying sufficient pressure
  - Ask patient to open fist, with hand still lifted
  - The hand will appear blanched
  - Release pressure over the ulnar artery
  - The normal colouration of the hand should return within 2–5 seconds
  - If it takes >7 seconds to return, this indicates insufficient ulnar artery blood supply to hands; in this situation, an ABG at the radial artery should be avoided.
- Blood pressure in both arms.

Head and neck

Inspect

Eyes
- Xanthalesma
- Corneal arcus.

Mouth
- Central cyanosis.

Palpate
- Carotid pulse – character and volume.

Auscultate
- Carotid bruit.

Axilla

Inspect and palpate
- Scars – with iliac disease an axillofemoral bypass is performed by taking a graft from the axillary artery to the femoral vessels. Palpate for the graft down the side of the chest.

Chest
- Median sternotomy scar – coronary artery bypass graft (CABG).

Abdomen

Inspect

- Pulsation
- Scar:
  - Midline laparotomy for emergency abdominal aortic aneurysm (AAA) repair and any aortobifemoral bypass
  - Transverse abdominal incision for an elective AAA repair.

Palpate

- Abdominal aorta:
  - Pulsatile and expansatile mass above the umbilicus indicates AAA
  - If only pulsatile and not expansile it is a transmitted pulse, which is normal
  - Attempt to feel for an iliac and femoral aneurysm if AAA is felt.

Iliac artery runs obliquely from the bifurcation of aorta at L1/L2 Diagonally across the abdomen. External iliac artery passes under the inguinal ligament becoming the Femoral artery. The femoral pulse is located at the mid-inguinal point, which lies midway between the symphysis pubis and the anterior superior iliac spine.

Auscultate

For bruits:

- Iliac artery
- Aorta
- Renal artery.

Legs

Inspect

- Surgical scars:
  - Long scar on medial calf for CABG
  - Vertical scar over mid-inguinal ligament – indicates bypass graft for femoral artery and for femoral embolectomy.
  - Midline laparotomy scar plus two vertical scars for aortobifemoral bypass graft
  - Varicose veins scars – located at the saphenofemoral junction found 4 cm lateral and inferior to the pubic tubercle; usually 3–4 mm in diameter
- Colour – white, blue/purple, black
- Tropic skin changes
- Ulceration and gangrene
- Amputations
- Hair distribution.
- Muscle wasting
- Coexistent venous disease (preferably whilst standing).

> ### Colour meanings
>
> **White:** ischaemia
>
> **Blue or purple:** venous insufficiency
>
> **Black:** gangrene

> ### Ulceration properties
>
> - **Venous ulcer** – typically in "gaiter" area over medial calf. Slopped edges. Look for haemosiderin deposition, lipodermatosclerosis (thin tight shiny skin) and visible varicose veins or previous scars from varicose vein surgery
>
> - **Arterial ulcer** – painful punched out ulcer (vertical edges), necrosis (black) with absent pulses, inspect between toes, under the heel.
>
> - **Neuropathic ulcer** – painless ulcer within pressure area (e.g., sole of foot) with reduced sensation. Typically in diabetics.
>
> - **Mixed ulcers** – mixed features.

Palpate

- Temperature of legs and feet – feel bilaterally with back of hands
- Capillary refill time (CRT):
  - Press on toe nailbed for 5 seconds
  - Release pressure
  - Note time taken for blanching to disappear
  - More than 2 seconds means adequate peripheral circulation
  - Avoid pressing on nail bed if evidence of digital ulceration; can press over the skin of a distal phalanx instead
- Swelling, particularly at the calves and ankles (pretibial/pitting oedema)
- Muscle atrophy, particularly of the quadriceps; determined by measuring and comparing the circumference of both thighs, at a fixed distance above the knee
- Peripheral pulses on both sides:
  - Dorsalis pedis – ask the patient to dorsiflex the foot, and extend the toes. The pulse is found in the groove just lateral to the extensor hallucis longus tendon on the dorsum of the foot. Place all the finger tips of one hand in this groove, until the pulse is palpable
  - Posterior tibial – located in the groove between the medial malleolus and tendocalcaneus (Achilles' tendon). Place two fingers in this groove
  - Popliteal pulse, bimanual palpation – ask the patient to relax, flex the knee slightly and press your fingertips into the popliteal fossa, applying counter-pressure with your thumb at the front of the knee. Remember the artery is located deep in the popliteal

fossa, and is normally difficult to feel. Consider a popliteal aneurysm if the popliteal pulse is easy to feel!

- Femoral pulse – found half way between ASIS and pubic symphysis, just below the inguinal ligament; the so-called mid-inguinal point. Press with two fingers, may be easier to palpate with leg abducted and externally rotated at hip
- Aortofemoral delay
- Grade pulses – absent, weak, normal, increased, bounding
- Palpate the carotids pulses bilaterally – don't palpate both at once
- Palpate the abdominal aorta.

Special manoeuvres

Buerger's test

- Patient starts in supine position, legs resting horizontally
- Holding on to both legs, gradually raise them upwards, noting any change in colouration of either foot
- The best place to look for any change of colour is the toes
- The angle of elevation at which the toes of a limb begin to develop pallor defines the vascular angle/ Buerger's angle for that limb
- A limb with sufficient arterial supply rises to 90 degrees without any change in colour; the toes maintain their pink/ normal colouration
- A limb with a severe reduction of arterial blood supply may have Buerger's angle less than 20 degrees

Dependence test

After conducting Buerger's test, the patient's legs should be placed in a dependent position: ideally the patient should sit with their legs hanging over the edge of the bed.

- Note the time taken for the normal pink colouration to return to the toes
- This should normally take no more than 10 seconds
- More than 10 seconds capillary filling time indicates some degree of arterial obstruction; 15–30 seconds indicates severe obstruction
- If toes turn purple/ crimson, this indicates severe ischaemia (reactive hyperaemia).

Auscultate

- Femoral bruit

Finishing off

- Thank the patient
- Ask if they need any help getting dressed
- Wash hands
- Present findings
- Summarise.

Mention that you would:

- Ask to see the results of ankle–brachial pressure index studies (see below) and/or digital subtraction angiography

- A full assessment of motor power and sensation, since reduction of leg strength is a manifestation of severe arterial deficiency, and sensory changes may be associated with various vascular conditions (diabetes)
- Repeat a vascular examination post exercise
- Examine the peripheral arterial system in the arms (see below)
- Perform a full cardiovascular examination.

ABPI (ankle: brachial pressure index)

Measured using Doppler probe (to detect blood flow as above) and standard blood pressure cuff

A: determine the pressure needed to occlude blood flow (systolic pressure) in the brachial artery at the arm

B: determine the pressure needed to occlude blood flow (systolic pressure) in the ankle arteries (dorsalis pedis or posterior tibial)

ABPI = **B** divided by **A**

Interpretation:

Normal ABPI > 1.0

ABPI < 0.9	some degree of arterial occlusion in leg
ABPI 0.3–0.6	severe arterial occlusion
ABPI < 0.3	*critical limb ischaemia* (gangrene, ulceration)

Varicose Veins Examination

Examiners instructions

"Please examine this patient's varicose veins and present your findings."

Common OSCE cases

- Primary varicose veins – usually saphenofemoral incompetence causing long saphenous varicose veins
- Secondary varicose veins – usually due to pelvic mass (e.g., tumour or pregnancy) or DVT
- Thread veins

Key signs associated with common OSCE cases

- **Primary varicose veins:** occur in long saphenous vein distribution (medial thigh and calf) usually due to saphenofemoral incompetence. Short saphenous varicose veins occur below knee laterally and are due to saphenopopliteal incompetence.

- **Secondary varicose veins:** usually due to pelvic mass (e.g., tumour or pregnancy) or DVT. Ensure you examine the abdomen of any patient with varicose veins and ask about a history of deep venous thrombosis.

- **Thread veins:** tiny superficial dilated veins within the skin.

Wh   Wash hands

I   Introduce yourself and identify patient

S   Summarise how you would examine the legs

P   Permission

E   Expose both legs keeping underwear on

R   Reposition standing up

S   State of patient (well/unwell, pregnant)

     Signs around bed – TED stockings

ACE TIPS

- Ask the patient if they are in any pain before you touch them

- Ask specifically about hip and back pain before you move them

Patient standing

It is wise to ask the patient to stand if the instruction from the examiner is to "examine the legs", as you will have to determine whether they want you to perform a venous or an arterial examination. You can ask for clarification, but they may not always tell you. Getting the patient to stand whilst suitably exposed may give the game away.

Inspect

- Scars
- Asymmetry
- Deformity
- Distribution of varicose veins:
    - Medial thigh – long saphenous varicose veins extending up to saphenofemoral junction
    - Back of knee – short saphenous varicose veins extending up to saphenopopliteal junction
    - Medial calf – calf perforators
- Look especially for:
    - Venous ulcers – typically sloped ulcers within gaiter area over medial calf, starting around medial malleolus
    - Venous eczema
    - Haemosiderosis
    - Lipodermatosclerosis – a triad of haemosiderin deposition, induration and fibrosis. Legs have an inverted champagne bottle appearance
    - Saphena varix – this is a dilatation where the great saphenous vein meets the femoral vein. It is found approximately 4 cm below and lateral to the pubic tubercle and may have a cough impulse. May be confused with a femoral hernia!

Palpate

- Ask if the veins are painful before you touch them
- Run hand along path of the long and short saphenous vein and the surrounding tributaries.
- Feel for:
    - Distendended veins
    - Tenderness
    - Hardening of skin

Special manoeuvres

- Cough impulse:
    - Feel over the saphenofemoral junction
    - Ask patient to cough.
    - Feel for thrill
    - Repeat manoeuvre at the saphenopopliteal junction
- Tap test:
    - Place fingers at lower end of a varicose vein
    - Tap an upper section of the same vein
    - Feel for a percussion impulse.

Patient lying

Torniquet test

Identifies the location of incompetence beneath the saphenofemoral junction.

- Elevate leg to empty distended veins, "milk" the veins empty. Be gentle, as you don't want to hurt the patient
- Tie tourniquet high up around the upper thigh below saphenofemoral junction
- Ask patient to stand up
- Look for filling of the veins below tourniquet
- If the lower veins fill, this indicates valvular incompetence below the tourniquet
- If the lower veins do not fill, remove the tourniquet
- Look again for filling of veins
- If these veins fill, this indicates valvular incompetence at the site of the tourniquet.

Repeat manoeuvre moving tourniquet down the leg to identify the site of valvular incompetence.

Trendelenburg test

Identifies whether there is incompetence at the saphenofemoral junction

- Elevate leg to empty distended veins
- Milk the veins empty – they will visibly gutter
- Place fingers firmly over the saphenofemoral junction
- Ask patient to stand up
- If the lower veins do not fill until you release your fingers this indicates saphenofemoral vein incompetence.

Perthes' test

Identifies if there is deep venous insufficiency e.g., an old undetected DVT.

- Identify the level of incompetence using the tourniquet
- Wrap the tourniquet at the site of incompetence
- Ask patient to bounce up and down on their tip toes to work the calf pump
- If the leg swells, turns blue and is painful, there is deep venous insufficiency.

Finishing off

- Thank patient
- Cover them up
- Wash hands
- Present findings
- Summarise.

Mention that you would:

- Examine the abdomen for a abdominal pelvic mass causing obstruction to the IVC
- Perform rectal examination
- Perform pelvic examination in females
- Examine external genitalia in males.

Case presentation

"In summary this lady has varicose veins bilaterally in the medial aspect of the calves. These veins do not extend past the popliteal fossa. She also has associated skin changes in the form of venous eczema. She has scars on the right leg medial aspect indicating previous varicose vein surgery. She also has haemosiderin deposition over the gaiter areas of both legs."

ACE TIP

Patients with varicose veins are easy to find for OSCE examinations, and are therefore very common surgical OSCE cases. The examination routine is simple and practicing will ensure good marks in this station.

ACE TIPS

- Varicose veins can be primary or secondary (caused by pelvic masses obstructing the sapheno-femoral junction e.g. tumours, pregnancy and occurring post deep vein thrombosis).

- Complications of varicose veins (bleeding, thrombophlebitis, venous eczema and ulceration).

- Management is:

  - Conservative – graduated compression stockings

  - Medical – injection with sclerosant such as sodium tetradecyl sulphate

  - Surgical – ligation of incompetent saphenofemoral junction or saphenopopliteal junction or incompetent perforator, often followed by surgical stripping of long saphenous vein and avulsion of smaller veins. Endovenous laser ablation of varicose veins is increasing in popularity as a minimally invasive alternative.

Investigations

- Venous duplex ultrasound
- Blood tests – coagulation studies.

Section III
Specialities

◉ Hip Examination

Examiner's instruction

"Please examine this patient's hip."

Common OSCE cases

- Primary osteoarthritis (OA) of the hip
- Rheumatoid arthritis (RA) of the hip
- Avascular necrosis (AVN) of the hip
- Postoperative hip (total hip replacement, hip resurfacing hemiarthroplasty, dynamic hip screw)

Key signs associated with common OSCE cases

Most patients with hip pathology will demonstrate the following features:

- Antalgic gait (see text)

- Positive Trendelenburg's sign (see text)

- Reduction in range of motion – reduction in internal and external rotation is often the earliest sign of degenerative osteoarthritis of the hip.

Rheumatoid arthritis – to differentiate RA and OA, look for the distribution of arthritis in the hands.

Avascular necrosis of the hip – in advanced cases there will be reduction in range of motion especially internal rotation with the hip in flexion. The diagnosis is mainly based on the history and radiological investigations (see below for key radiological features of AVN).

Post-operative hips – look for tell-tale surgical scars over the hip, and be sure to check posteriorly for scars.

Wh Wash hands
I Introduce yourself and identify patient
S Summarise how you would like to examine their hips – standing, walking and lying
P Permission
E Expose the leg keeping underwear on
R Reposition patient standing
S State of patient – well/unwell, ability to move
     Signs around bed – walking aids.

Stand at the end of the bed and look at the patient

ACE TIPS

Ask the patient if they are in any pain before you touch them

Patient standing

Inspect

- Scars
- Asymmetry
  - Front – pelvic tilting, quadriceps wasting
  - Side – normal lumbar lordosis
  - Behind – gluteal wasting
- Deformity

Palpate

Trendelenburg test

- Manoeuvre – place hands on anterior superior iliac spines (ASIS), and ask patient to lift *right leg* off floor and watch your hands:
  - Normal: your *left* hand should rise as the pelvis tilts
  - Explanation: this tilt is brought about by contraction of the patient's left hip abductors
- Positive Trendelenburg (abnormal): left hand falls as pelvis tilts
  - Explanation: left hip abductors are not working properly
- Mnemonic: "the sound side sags"
- Repeat on the other side.

Patient walking

Ask patient to walk to end of room and back to assess gait:

- Antalgic – less time is spent on the painful leg while walking, which shows as a shortened stance phase in the gait cycle
- Trendelenburg – waddling
- High-stepping – foot-drop

What is the gait cycle?

1. Stance phase
2. Toe off phase
3. Swing phase
4. Heel strike

Patient lying

Examine the good hip first then the bad one to compare the two.

Inspect

Apparent and real leg lengths:

- Manoeuvre – measure distance from xiphisternum to tip of each medial malleolus
  - Unequal length may be either a *true* or *apparent* difference

- Manoeuvre – to differentiate measure distance from ASIS to tip of medial malleolus to give true leg length
  - Explanation:
    - If the true lengths are the same, this suggests an apparent leg length discrepancy, e.g., pelvic tilting, muscle contractures, scoliosis
    - If the true lengths are different, there is a bony difference in either the femur, tibia or both.

Palpate

- Feel over greater trochanter for tenderness.

Move

Hip flexion

- Passively flex patients hip to upper limit.
- Normal – 120 degrees
- Is limitation due to pain or stiffness?

Thomas' test – fixed flexion deformity

- Place your left hand under the patient's lumbar spine.
- Bring patient's knee up towards their chest with your right hand.
- Once the hip has reached its maximal flexion further movement towards the chest can still occur by tilting of the pelvis but this will flatten the lumbar lordosis, which you will feel with your left hand.
- If, as you flatten the lordosis, the patient's *other* thigh starts to lift off the couch this suggests a fixed flexion deformity.
- Repeat on the other side.

Hip extension (10–15 degrees)

- Ask the patient to lie prone and lift their leg up to the ceiling.

Internal rotation/external rotation (45 degrees)

- Flex right hip and knee to 90 degrees.
- Steady knee with your left hand and rotate hip with your right hand holding the patient's foot.
- Repeat with left leg.

Note: moving the foot towards the midline is external hip rotation and away is internal hip rotation.

Abduction/adduction (40 degrees/25 degrees respectively)

- Place your left arm across the patient's pelvis (on the ASIS) to ensure pelvis is not tilting during the examination.
- Hold patient's lower leg in right hand and move foot away from the midline.
- Note degree of abduction at which the pelvis starts to tilt.
- Now move the foot across the midline to measure adduction.
- Repeat with the other leg.

Finishing off

- Thank the patient
- Make sure patient is comfortable and offer to help cover them up
- Wash hands
- Present and consider age of patient in forming differential
- Summarise.

Mention that you would:

Rheumatoid arthritis (RA) versus primary osteoarthritis (OA) of the hip

- RA typically symmetrical polyarthritis

- Look for the distribution of arthritis in the hands

- RA association with extra-articular manifestations

- Rheumatoid factor +ve in 70–80% of RA; –ve in OA

- ESR and CRP frequently elevated in RA

- Perform a full neurovascular examination of lower limbs – including femoral pulses
- Examine lumbar spine and knee (joint above and below)
- Plain radiographs of hip.

Investigations

Primary osteoarthritis of the hip

- Radiographs – two views AP pelvis and lateral of the hip.

Avascular necrosis of the hip

- Radiographs (see box)
- MRI (early changes are of bone marrow ischaemia)
- Bone scan (increased uptake)
- Single photon emission computed tomography (SPECT) scan.

Radiographic findings in AVN of the hip

- Normal in the early stages

- Osteopoenia and sclerosis develops

- Later subchondral collapse results giving the characteristic "crescent sign"

- Secondary osteoarthritis changes

RA of the hip

- Rheumatoid factor (positive in 70–80%)
- Increased inflammatory markers (ESR, CRP).

Common hip operations

- **A total hip replacement:** replacing the acetabulum with an acetabular cup prosthesis, and the femoral head and neck is replaced with a femoral prosthesis with a stem that extends into the femoral shaft.

- **Hip resurfacing:** replacing the acetabulum with an acetabular cup, the femoral neck is preserved and the femoral head is "resurfaced" with a prosthesis.

- **A hip hemiarthroplasty:** often used in treating intracapsular fractured neck of femurs, involves replacing the femoral head and neck with a femoral prosthesis. The acetabular side is not replaced.

- **A dynamic hip screw:** often used in treating inter-trochanteric fractured neck of femurs, involves a screw going into the femoral head attached to a plate secured with screws on the femoral shaft.

⦿ Knee Examination

Examiner's instruction

"Examine this patient's knee and present your finding."

Common OSCE cases

- Knee osteoarthritis (OA)
- Anterior cruciate ligament (ACL) injury
- Meniscal tears

Key signs associated with common OSCE cases

Knee osteoarthritis (OA): crepitus with decreased range of movement. Note any varus or valgus deformity. Varus deformity in patients with knee OA suggests narrowing of the joint space in the medial compartment of the knee.

Anterior cruciate ligament (ACL) injuries: usually a young male patient with a football or skiing injury. Anterior draw test with the knee flexed to 90 degrees, grasp the tibia and pull anteriorly – anterior translation suggests an ACL tear.

Medial/lateral meniscal tears: palpation along the medial and lateral joint lines with the knee flexed at 90 degrees will cause tenderness in patients with meniscal tears. McMurray's test (see text) causes pain and occasionally clicking on the affected side in a meniscal tear.

Wh Wash hands
I Introduce yourself and identify patient
S Summarise how you would like to examine their knee – standing, walking and lying
P Permission
E Expose the leg keeping underwear on
R Reposition patient standing
S State of patient (well/unwell), ability to move
Signs around bed – walking aids.

Stand at the end of the bed and look at the patient

ACE TIPS

Ask the patient if they are in any pain before you touch them

Patient standing

Inspect

From the front

- Scars
- Asymmetry

- Deformity – varus (bow leg) or valgus (knock knees)
- Specific:
  - skin changes (erythema/psoriasis, etc.)
  - swelling (bursae/effusion/cysts)
  - quadriceps wasting.

From the back:
- Specific – popliteal swelling (Baker's cyst).

Move
- Ask patient to walk to end of room and back – antalgic gait/use of walking aid.

Patient lying
Examine the good knee first then the bad one and compare the two.

Feel
- Quadriceps wasting – measure circumference
- Warmth – use the back of the hands to compare warmth over knee to thigh
- Joint line:
  - Flex the knee to 90 degrees
  - Feel along joint line for tenderness/swelling.

The joint line path
Begin at the femoral condyles and move to the base of the patella, travel down the patella tendon towards the tibial tuberosity.
Effusion:
- Patellar tap (larger effusion)
  - Place left hand on anterior thigh, sweep distally up to patella. This empties any fluid down from the suprapatellar pouch
  - Tap the patella using right thumb listening for a clunk
- Sweep test (smaller effusion)
  - Sweep the right hand up medial aspect of knee from distal to proximal
  - Continue up lateral side in same direction
  - Observe the hollow on the medial side for any fluid being pushed across
- Popliteal swellings
  - Slide both hands under the knee joint into the popliteal fossa
  - Feel for any swellings.

Move
- Fixed flexion deformity
  - Extend legs, place hands behind each knee.
  - Ask patient to maximally extend both knees
  - The normal knee will push against the hand

- If it is abnormal, lift the opposite heel:
  - If deformity persists it is a flexion deformity
  - If knee is now fully straight it is an extensor lag
- Active
  - Ask patient to flex each knee and comment on the range – are they limited by pain or stiffness
- Passive
  - Support the weight of patients leg by their heel
  - Place your other hand on the surface of the patella
  - Flex the knee:
    - Comment on the range
    - Feel for crepitus.

Special manoeuvres

Anterior drawer test

Testing for laxity of the anterior cruciate ligament.

First inspect from the side whilst the patient's knees are flexed looking for a posterior sag of the tibia. If this is present it indicates a posterior cruciate tear and you would get a false positive anterior draw test.

- Grip the upper tibia with both hands, thumbs on the tuberosity and fingers behind
- Feel hamstrings ensure they are relaxed
- Sit on the patient's feet for stability
- Pull the tibia firmly towards you looking for any significant movement.

Lachman's test

This may also be performed to assess ACL pathology.

- With the knee flexed 15–30 degrees, grasp the femur with one hand and the tibia with the other.
- Keeping the femur stable, pull the tibia anteriorly.
- Anterior translocation of the tibia on the femur is seen in anterior cruciate ligament tears.

McMurray's test

Now turn to your examiners telling them that you would like to perform McMurray's test for meniscal pathology, but that you understand it can be painful and would they like you to proceed?

- Lateral meniscal tear
  - Place left hand on the knee joint
  - Flex the knee to 90 degrees
  - Invert the patients foot and support the heel
  - Extend the knee feeling for a click
- Medial meniscal tear
  - Place left hand on the knee joint
  - Evert the patients foot and support the heel

- Flex the knee to 90 degrees
- Extend the knee feeling for a click – positive McMurray's test
- Collateral ligament stability (for right leg)
  - Support distal tibia in right hand, support behind outer aspect of knee with left hand
    - Apply a valgus strain to the distal tibia
    - Assess laxity of medial collateral ligament
  - Support behind inner aspect of knee with left hand
    - Apply a varus strain to the distal tibia
    - Assess laxity of lateral collateral ligament.

Finishing off
- Thank the patient
- Make sure patient is comfortable and offer to help cover them up
- Wash hands
- Present and consider age of patient in forming differential
- Summarise.

Mention that you would:
- Examine the hips and ankles
- Full neurovascular examination of lower limbs
- Inspect plain radiographs of the knee.

Effusions

- In meniscus injuries – the effusion is small/moderate and develops several hours/days after the injury.

- In ACL injuries – the effusion is large and often occurs within a few hours after the injury.

Investigations
Knee osteoarthritis
- Plain radiographs – AP (standing), lateral and skyline views.

Anterior cruciate ligament injuries
- Plain radiographs – views as above for knee OA. May show fracture of tibial spine, usually normal.
- MRI.

Meniscal tears
- Plain radiographs, usually normal
- MRI.

⚙ Shoulder Examination

Examiner's instruction

"Please examine this patient's shoulders."

Common OSCE cases

- Subacromial impingement
- Rotator cuff tears
- Frozen shoulder
- Glenohumeral osteoarthritis (OA)
- Acromioclavicular joint OA
- Recurrent dislocation

Key signs of common OSCE cases

Subacromial impingement: painful arc – pain in the arc of abduction between 60 and 120 degrees. Neer's impingement test: Stand behind the patient, stabilise their scapula with one hand and hold their forearm with the other. With the shoulder in internal rotation (point thumb down to the floor) passively elevate the arm in abduction.

Rotator cuff tears: difficulty in initiating abduction is suggestive of a supraspinatus rotator cuff tear (traumatic in the younger patient/secondary to chronic impingement in the older patient). The tests for rotator cuff muscle power are described below.

Frozen shoulder: pain is felt near deltoid insertion. There is marked reduction throughout all range of motion, especially passive external rotation.

Osteoarthritis: with one hand resting over the shoulder, abduct the arm with your other hand feeling for crepitus during the movement. Try and locate the source of the crepitus to either the acromioclavicular joint (ACJ) or glenohumeral joint. Pain from ACJ OA produces pain at the extremes of range of elevation in abduction or flexion. Pain radiating to the back of the shoulder suggests glemohumeral involvement.

Recurrent dislocation: the anterior apprehension test: standing behind the patient (seated) abduct their shoulder to 90 degrees then slowly externally rotate the shoulder with one hand while pushing the head of the humerus gently anteriorly with the other. If the patient has instability they will feel apprehension or refuse to continue *(do not use any force as it is possible to dislocate the shoulder in this setting).*

Wh Wash hands

I Introduce yourself and identify patient

S Summarise how you would like to examine their shoulder

P Permission

E Expose shoulders keeping underwear on.

R   Reposition patient standing

S   State of patient (well/unwell).

Inspect

* Scars, skin changes
* Asymmetry
    - Front – deltoid wasting, effusion
    - Behind – trapezius wasting, rotator cuff wasting
* Deformity
    - Clavicle
    - Winging of the scapula – ask patient to push against wall.

Palpate

* Begin at the sternoclavicular joint moving along the clavicle from medial to lateral
* Move laterally to the acromioclavicular joint
* Travel over the acromion towards the spine of the scapula
* Continue on towards the medial border
* Palpate down to the tip of the medial border of the scapula
* Journey up the lateral border to reach the shoulder joint
* Move across lateral border of shoulder joint to end at the acromioclavicular joint
* Watch the patient's face throughout to assess for tenderness, and feel for any deformity.

Move

* Start by examining the range of motion of the cervical spine to rule out shoulder pain radiating from painful neck movements:
    * Flexion – ask patient to touch their chin to their chest
    * Extension – ask patient to look up to the ceiling
    * Lateral rotation – (normal 80 degrees) ask patient to turn their head to look over one shoulder then the other
    * Lateral flexion – (normal 40 degrees) ask patient to lower their ear to their shoulder and repeat on the other side.
* Shoulder movements – start with active movements (the patient moves) and repeat the movements passively (you move the patient)
    * Flexion – (normal 170 degrees) ask patient to elevate straight arm anteriorly
    * Extension – (normal is 60 degrees) ask patient to swing straight arms posteriorly
    * Abduction – (normal range 170 degrees) begin with straight arm by side and palm facing forwards, ask patient to raise arm out to the side.
    * Adduction – (normal range 50 degrees) begin with elbow flexed to 90 degrees with forearm resting across the upper abdomen, ask patient to bring arm medially across the body
    * External rotation – (normal range is 60 degrees) begin with elbows flexed to 90 degrees with palms facing medially, keeping the elbow fixed by their sides, ask patient to move forearm outwards

- Internal rotation – (normal is approximately T7 corresponding to the tip of the scapula) ask patient to extend shoulders and flex elbows to reach behind their back (as if to do up a brastrap) and record highest vertebral level that the patient's thumb can reach.

Special tests

- **Rotator cuff integrity** (pain, weakness or inability to do these movements suggest tears):

  - Supraspinatus – ask patient to abduct from 0 to 30 degrees against resistance

  - Infraspinatus/teres minor – test external rotation (as described above) against resistance

  - Subscapularis – stand behind the patient, ask them to place their hands behind them with the dorsum resting against the lower back, ask them to lift their hand off their back against resistance.

- **Neer's impingement test**, as described in the box *"Key signs of common OSCE cases"*. The original Neer's test involved instilling local anaesthetic into the subacromial space and repeating the manoeuvre. If the pain is abolished the test is positive.

- **The anterior apprehension test**, as described in the box *"Key signs of common OSCE cases"*. Shoulder instability can be anterior, posterior or a combination of these. The commonest dislocation is an anterior dislocation. The posterior apprehension test is done with the patient lying supine with the arm flexed to 90 degrees in internal rotation. Apply a posterior force along the humerus from the elbow. This will make the patient with posterior instability apprehensive.

Finishing off

- Thank patient
- Cover them up
- Wash hands
- Present and consider age of patient in forming differential
- Summarise.

Mention that you would:

- Perform a full neurovascular examination of the upper limb
- Examine the cervical spine
- Look at plain radiographs of the shoulder.

Investigations

Subacromial impingement

- Radiographs – at least two views, AP and axillary views of the shoulder (usually normal in early stages, may show subchondral cysts and sclerosis of the greater tuberosity where the cuff inserts)

- In chronic cases or where rotator cuff tears are suspected, investigations are as follows for rotator cuff pathology.

Rotator cuff pathology

- Radiographs – AP and axillary views of the shoulder (loss of space between humerus and acromion, glenohumeral or acromioclavicular joint osteoarthritis)
- USS (may show complete tears but is operator dependent)
- MRI (useful for complete tears)
- Shoulder arthroscopy.

Glenohumeral and acromioclavicular joint osteoarthritis

- Radiographs – AP and axillary views of the shoulder. Look for the typical radiological changes in OA in the respective joints: joint space narrowing, osteophyte formation, and subchondral cysts.

Frozen shoulder

- Diagnosed mainly from history and examination. Radiographs are taken to rule out glenohumeral OA and shoulder dislocation.

Shoulder instability

- Radiographs – to rule out Bankart lesion (avulsion of the anteroinferior glenoid labrum) or Hill-Sachs lesion (posterolateral indentation of the humeral head from anterior dislocation)
- CT or MRI
- Shoulder arthroscopy
- Examination under anaesthesia – to determine direction of instability

Spine Examination

Examiner's instruction

"This patient complains of back pain. Examine this patient's spine and present your findings."

Common OSCE cases
- Ankylosing spondylitis
- Prolapsed intervertebral disc
- Spinal stenosis

Key signs in differentiating OSCE cases

Ankylosing spondylitis: affects mainly the spine and sacroiliac joints. The patient is usually male aged between 15 and 25 years. There is decreased range of motion in the spine especially extension. Perform the "wall test" – ask the patient to stand with his back against a wall, the occiput, scapulae, buttocks and heels should all touch the wall. Patients with ankylosing spondylitis will be unable to do this. Chest expansion is markedly decreased.

Prolapsed intervertebral disc:

- Positive straight leg raise test – assesses disk prolapse at L5/S1 with sciatic nerve root irritation. When lying supine with knee extended hold foot with one hand and lift leg straight up until patient experiences pain in buttocks radiating *below* the knee, estimate angle of elevation. Lower the leg to relieve discomfort and dorsiflex the foot – this reproduces the discomfort (the Lasegue test).

- Femoral stretch test when lying prone – assess for pain in the thigh indicating a positive femoral stretch test, i.e., an L4 radiculopathy mostly due to L4/L5 disc herniation.

Spinal stenosis: examination findings are generally non-specific. There is often pain in lumbar extension, sensory changes in the lower limbs, and weakness of toe extension.

Wh Wash hands

I Introduce yourself and identify patient

S Summarise how you would like to examine their spine – standing, walking and lying.

P Permission

E Expose upper body keeping underwear on; equipment – measuring tape

R Reposition patient standing

S State of patient (well/unwell), ability to move.

Patient standing and walking

Inspect

* Scars, skin changes
* Asymmetry
  - Side – kyphosis, hyperlordosis, loss of lumber lordosis
  - Behind – scoliosis, tapezius wasting
* Deformity
* Gait – ask patient to walk to end of room and back
* Measure wall–occiput distance if appropriate (if ankylosing spondylitis?).

Palpate

* Begin at the uppermost palpable cervical vertebrae (C7)
* Gently feel down each vertebral spinous process for tenderness and deformity
* At the lumber base travel out to feel both sacroiliac joints
* Return to the cervical region to palpate down the paravertebral muscles on either side.

Move

Cervical

* Flexion – bend neck forwards
* Extension – tilt head back
* Rotation – turn head to each side
* Lateral flexion – bring ear down to shoulder.

Thoracic

* Rotation:
  - Place your hands on patient's iliac crests to fix pelvis
  - Ask patient to cross arms over chest and twist around looking over their shoulder.

Lumbar

* Flexion:
  - Shober's test:
    * Mark out dimple of Venus
    * Identify two consecutive vertebrae 10 cm above
    * Ask patient to flex, and measure the increase in distance between two points – normal is more than 5 cm.
  - Alternatively, place two fingers on consecutive vertebrae
  - Ask patient to bend forwards and assess separation of fingers
* Extension
  - Keep fingers on the vertebrae
  - Ask patient to lean backwards without bending knees
  - Assess closure of fingers

* Lateral flexion
  - Begin with patient's arms by their side, ask patient to bend and slide hands sideways as far down leg as possible
  - Describe level they can reach.

Patient lying

* Femoral stretch test when lying prone:
  * "Is the pain in your hip or your thigh?"
  * Pain in the thigh indicates a positive femoral stretch test, i.e., an L4 radiculopathy mostly due to L4/L5 disc herniation.
* Straight leg raise when lying supine:
* Pain – sciatic nerve root irritation in buttocks radiating below the knee indicates a positive straight leg raise, i.e., L5/S1 radiculopathy mostly due to L5/S1 disc herniation.
  * Hold patient's foot with one hand and raise leg
  * Estimate angle of elevation.

Finishing off

* Thank patient
* Cover them up
* Wash hands
* Present and consider age of patient in forming differential
* Summarise.

Mention that you would:

* Full neurological examination of upper and lower limbs
* Look for the following if you were presented with an ankylosing spondylitis patient:
  * Anterior uveitis
  * Aortitis
  * Aortic regurgitation
  * Apical pulmonary fibrosis
  * Amyloidosis
  * Achilles tendonitis.

Case presentation

"This is a middle aged gentleman who experiences symptoms of pain and stiffness throughout his spine. He has grossly reduced movements in the cervical, thoracic and lumber spine. He has an increased occiput distance. All these findings tie in with a diagnosis of ankylosing spondylosis".

Investigations

Ankylosing spondylitis

* Blood tests
  * Inflammatory markers are raised
  * HLA-B27 is present in the majority of cases

- Radiographs – AP and lateral of the spine. Lumbar spine AP will show the cardinal sign of sacroiliac joint erosion later progressing to ankylosis (fusion of the joint). The vertebrae become squared off. Syndesmophytes (bony bridges) form between the vertebra and lead to the appearance of a "bamboo spine".

Prolapsed intervertebral discs

- Radiographs – AP and lateral of the lumbar spine (not usually helpful though may show disc space narrowing, osteophyte formation)
- MRI – the investigation of choice. Disc prolapse occur most commonly at L4–5 and L5–S1 levels.

Spinal stenosis

- Radiographs – AP and lateral of the spine to exclude spinal deformities (e.g., scoliosis) or other pathological process of the spine (e.g., infection or tumour)
- MRI – the preferred imaging test to diagnose spinal stenosis
- CT-myelography – invasive due to injection of contrast, though its use has decreased with the use of MRI

◉ GALS Screen

GALS examination is a screening examination looking at the appearance and movement of the joints in gait, arms, legs and spine.

Wh Wash hands

I Introduce yourself and identify patient

S Summarise that you would like to examine the function of their joints

P Permission

E Expose all joints by asking patient to undress to underpants; equipment – measuring tape

R Reposition asking patient to stand

S State of patient (well/unwell), able to stand or not. Any clues around the bed, e.g., walking stick, frame etc.

Always begin by asking the three important questions:

1. Do you have any pain or stiffness in any of your joints, muscles or back?

2. Do you have any difficulty walking up and down stairs?

3. Do you have any difficulty dressing or bathing yourself?

Patient standing

Inspect

- Abnormal posture
- Deformities
- Swellings
- Scars.

Gait

Ask the patient to walk to the other side of room and back.

Inspect

- Symmetry of movement
- Antalgic gait, waddling, festinant/shuffling (Parkinson's disease), wide based (cerebellar ataxia), high stepping (foot drop) etc.
- Arm swing.

Spine

Inspect

From behind with patient standing:

- Spinal deformities, e.g., abnormal kyphosis, lordosis, scoliosis
- Asymmetry
- Scars

* Level iliac crests
* Muscle wasting, e.g., shoulder, thigh, calves.

Movement

Ask the patient to:

* Touch their ear to their shoulder without moving shoulder up, and repeat on other side (lateral cervical flexion)
* Bend forward and touch their toes (forward flexion). Before they do this, place one finger on a spinal process of a lumbar vertebrae and another finger on the spinal process of the adjacent lumbar vertebrae on patient's back. Record the degree of forward flexion by estimating the distance between both fingers during flexion. This is to identify reduced forward flexion, e.g., ankylosing spondylitis.

Arms

Inspect

* Muscle wasting
* Swellings
* Scars.

Movement

Ask the patient to:

* Raise their arms above their head and touch the backs of their neck with their thumbs (shoulder abduction and external rotation)
* Move their hands to try and touch their scapulae on their backs (shoulder adduction and internal rotation)
* Touch their shoulders (elbow flexion)
* Straighten elbows out in front (elbow extension)
* Place both hands together in the prayer position (wrist extension)
* Place both hands in the inverse prayer position touching both dorsum of hands (wrist flexion)
* Keep both elbows fixed at hips and move hands outwards from midline and towards the midline (elbow internal and external rotation)
* Put hands out in front with palms facing the ceiling, then turn both hands so that the palms are facing down to the floor (supination and pronation)
* Place both hands out with palms facing the floor and then squeeze the metacarpophalangeal joints bilaterally in turn and look for pain or grimace
* Touch their thumbs to each finger (opposition)
* Place both hands out with palms facing the ceiling and then place your finger in their palm and ask them to squeeze as hard as they can (grip power).

Legs

Inspect

* Varus/valgus deformities
* Foot deformities, e.g., high arch

* Muscle wasting
* Swellings especially popliteal fossa for popliteal cyst
* Scars.

Movement

Ask the patient to:

* Bend their knee as much as possible and then straighten leg again whilst placing your hand on patient's knee feeling for crepitus (knee flexion and extension)
* Move their bent knee to touch their chest (hip flexion)
* Raise their legs as high as they can then take their leg and whilst bending their knee place one hand on their knee and the other holding their leg just above their ankle. Perform passive internal and external rotation of their hips looking at the patient's face whilst performing these manoeuvres to look for pain or grimacing
* Move their feet down at the ankle joint and then move their feet up towards their head (flexion and extension at ankle joint)
* Place their legs flat on the bed and squeeze the patient's metatarsophalangeal joints for tenderness looking at the patients face.

Finishing off

* Thank patient
* Cover them up/make comfortable
* Wash hands
* Present findings
* Summarise.

Mention that you would:

* Like to examine more comprehensively any particular joint that you found was abnormal on GALS screen.

1 Examiners questions

"What are the common findings of osteoarthritis in the hands?"

Swellings of the distal interphalangeal (DIP) joints (Heberden's nodes), proximal interphalangeal nodes (Bouchard's nodes) and squaring of the hands as a result of subluxation of the first MCP joints.

"Which joints are commonly affected in rheumatoid arthritis?"

Swelling of the metacarpophalangeal (MCP) joints, proximal interphalangeal (PIPs) with sparing of the DIP joints. Wrist subluxation, Boutonniere and Swan neck deformities in the fingers, Z-thumb deformity, metatarsophalangeal (MTP) joints and knees.

"What are the extra-articular manifestations of rheumatoid arthritis?"

Anaemia of chronic disease, rheumatoid nodules, carpel tunnel syndrome, splenomegaly (Felty's syndrome), lymphadenopathy, pleural effusion, pleurisy, pulmonary fibrosis, Caplan's syndrome, episcleritis, scleritis, keratoconjunctivitis sicca, pericarditis, osteoporosis.

"What investigation would you do for a patient with rheumatoid arthritis prior to them going for surgery and why?"

Cervical spine radiograph to exclude atlantoaxial subluxation.

"What one investigation would you like to perform in this patient with ankylosing spondylitis and why?"

Radiograph with anteroposterior (AP) view of the sacroiliac joints and lateral view of the lumbar spine. To look for erosions and sclerosis in the sacroiliac joints which are the earliest changes in ankylosing spondylitis. "Bamboo spine" is a late finding found in severe disease and not the earliest finding as mistaken by many medical students.

"What are the extra-articular findings in ankylosing spondylitis?"

Apical fibrosis, aortic regurgitation, anterior uveitis, Achilles tendonitis.

"What is a Baker's cyst?"

Popliteal cyst found in osteoarthritis.

"What would you see on synovial aspirate microscopy from a patient with gout?"

Negatively birefringent uric acid crystals.

"What would you see on synovial aspirate microscopy from a patient with pseudogout?"

Positively birefringent rhomboid shaped calcium pyrophosphate crystals.

◉ The Pregnant Abdomen

Examiner's instruction

"Demonstrate how you would examine the abdomen of a pregnant woman on the mannequin. Address any conversation you would have with a pregnant woman to the mannequin."

Wh Wash hands

I Introduce yourself and identify patient

S Summarise how you would examine the abdomen in a pregnant patient – "I would like to perform an examination by gently feeling your abdomen. Although it may be a bit uncomfortable, it should not be painful."

P Permission and priority questions:
  - "Do you feel the need to empty your bladder?"
  - "A female chaperone will be present."

E Expose the abdomen – "Please could you lift your clothes to expose your abdomen?"

R Reposition to the supine position.

S State of patient (well/unwell?).

Performing the abdominal examination

> ### ACE TIP
>
> When examining always look at he patient's face so you can determine whether or not you are causing any discomfort. With the pregnant abdomen some degree of deep palpation is required. However if you palpate slowly flexing at your metacarpophalangeal joint rather than at your finger tips you will not cause your patient pain.

Inspect:
- Linea nigra
- Striae gravidarum
- Scars.

Palpation/auscultation
- There are 6 steps to cover – start with FH (fundal height) and finish with FH (fetal heart):
- FH: **fundal height** – hold your left hand over the xiphisternum and begin palpating downwards to detect the uterine fundus. With your right hand, place the tip of your tape measure at the fundus and measure to the pubis symphysis. This distance in cm (+/–2) should correlate with the gestational age.
- Determining the **number of fetuses and the lie** – keep your hands parallel to each other on either side of the abdomen. Press in firmly but gently with one hand while doing the same with the other hand on the opposite side. Gradually move downwards to determine

where the fetal back lies. You will describe the lie as longitudinal, transverse or oblique depending on the orientation of the fetal spine to the midline. The absence of a smooth dorsal contour may indicate that the fetus is lying occipitoposterior, i.e., looking up; while the presence of numerous fetal poles may indicate a multiple pregnancy. In the second and early third trimesters only a pelvic mass and no definite fetal poles are present.

- **Palpating the presenting part** – this can be determined using Polick's manoeuvre. This involves using the thumb and index finger of your right hand on each side of the presenting part in the suprapubic region and gently but deeply pressing them in towards each other until either a firm mass (cephalic presentation) or a soft mass (a breech presentation) is felt.

- **How many fifths (5ths)** – don't let the 5ths confuse you: just imagine the fetal head divided into fifths in a coronal plane. If you can feel all of the head, i.e., 5/5 abdominally, it is unengaged ie not in the pelvis. Similarly if you can feel most of the head abdominally (i.e., 3/5 or 4/5) it is either 2/5 or 1/5 engaged (i.e., partially engaged). The converse holds.

- **Fetal heart (FH) auscultation** – you have already determined on which side the fetal back lies. Listen to the FH with the sonicade/ pinnard in the abdominal area over the fetal scapulae.

Finishing off
- Thank patient
- Cover them up
- Wash hands
- Present findings
- Summarise.

Case presentation
"In summarizing my findings the fundal height is 33 cm, which coincides with the period of gestation. It is a singleton fetus in a longitudinal lie, cephalic presentation, 3 fifths palpable, with the foetal heart being regular."

Bimanual Vaginal Examination

Examiner's instruction

"Demonstrate how you would perform a bimanual vaginal examination on a patient using the mannequin. Address any conversation you would have with a patient to the mannequin."

Wh Wash hands

I Introduce yourself and identify patient

S Summarise how you would examine the vagina – "I would like to perform a vaginal examination by inserting two well-lubricated gloved fingers into your vagina up towards your womb. Although it may be a bit uncomfortable, it should not be painful."

P Permission and priority questions:
- Do you feel the need to empty your bladder?
- A female chaperone will be present.
- At times nurses can come into the room without knocking – would you like the door locked?

E Expose lower half of the body – "Please could you go behind the curtain and remove your trousers and underwear. There is a drape laid out for you to cover yourself with."

R Reposition to the modified lithotomy position with patient lying flat, head on one pillow – "Bring the heels of your feet towards your bottom and let your knees fall to the side."

S State of patient (well/unwell).

This examination should always begin with palpation of the abdomen. However the examiner will usually ask you to skip this due to time. If you are asked to perform this step, ensure you keep the external genitalia covered.

Inspect
Vulva
- Varicosities
- Ulcers
- Discharge and bleeding
- Abnormal hair distribution
- Scars
- Atrophy
- Lumps.

Palpate
- Entering the vagina:
  - Lubricate gloved index and middle finger of right hand
  - Use thumb and index finger of left hand to separate the labia

- Warn patient that you are about to examine the vagina
- Gently insert index and middle fingers through vaginal introitus
- Palpate along canal for any masses
- At the cervix assess:
  - Size, shape
  - Consistency – hard/soft
  - Os open/ closed
  - Mobility
  - Cervical excitation
- Assessing the uterus:
  - With your right hand push up onto the cervix and simultaneously with your left press down on the uterine fundus. Your aim is to feel the uterus between your hands, i.e., bimanually
  - Estimate uterine size, shape, consistency, position, mobility
  - Determine whether uterus is anteverted/ retroverted uterus
- At the adnexa:
  - Move fingers into left fornix
  - Move palmar surface of left hand into left iliac fossa
  - Ballot with left hand against right fingers
  - Assess size and shape of left ovary along with any other palpable adnexal structures
  - Sweep fingers into right fornix and repeat
  - Remove fingers and inspect glove for blood or discharge
  - Remove gloves.

Finishing off
- Thank patient
- Cover them up
- Wash hands.

Mention that you would:
- Perform a speculum examination
- Take a smear.

⊙ Cervical Smear Test

Examiner's instruction

"Demonstrate how you would perform a cervical smear on a patient using the mannequin. Address any conversation you would have with a patient to the mannequin."

Wh Wash hands

I Introduce yourself and identify patient

S Summarise how you would like to perform a smear test – "I would like perform a smear test by inserting a speculum into your vagina and gently sweeping some of the cells within your cervix. Although it may be a bit uncomfortable, it should not be painful."

P Permission and priority questions:
- "Do you feel the need to empty your bladder?
- "A female chaperone will be present."
- "At times nurses can come into the room without knocking – would you like the door locked?"

E Expose lower half of body – "Please could you go behind the curtain and remove your trousers and underwear. There is a drape laid out for you to cover yourself with."

Equipment:
- Cusco's speculum – choose appropriate size – small/ medium/ large
- KY jelly, slides or LBC (liquid-based cytology medium)
- nonsterile gloves
- fixative
- Ayres spatula
- Endocervical brush/ cytobrush
- Set up slide – use pencil to write name/ hospital no./ D.O.B./ date

R Reposition to the modified lithotomy position with patient lying flat, head on one pillow – "Bring the heels of your feet towards your bottom and let your knees fall to the side"

S State of patient (well/unwell).

> **ACE TIP**
>
> Ask the patient if they are comfortable or in pain before you touch them

Inspect

Vulva
- Varicosities
- Ulcers
- Discharge or bleeding
- Abnormal hair distribution

* Scars
* Lumps.

Perform smear

Prepare equipment

* Ensure light source give adequate visibility
* Put on gloves
* Warm speculum blades under warm water
* Apply jelly onto blades.

Insert speculum

* Warn patient you are about to insert speculum
* Use thumb and index finger of left hand to hold open labia
* Gently insert speculum with blades closed and handles horizontal
* Rotate the handle facing upwards – place left fingers between the screw and the pubic area to minimize discomfort
* Open blades and identify the cervix
* Lock blades open
* Assess cervix:
  * Size/ shape
  * Open/closed.

Taking the smear

* Insert Ayres spatula or cytobrush through speculum into the endocervical canal
* Rotate the spatula or brush 360 degrees clockwise and anticlockwise
* Remove spatula and scrape cell onto the pre-named slide thoroughly, and immediately apply fixative
* If using the cytobrush, was the brush in a container with approx 10 ml of liquid medium
* Unscrew speculum
* Gently withdraw speculum a few centimetres keeping blades open manually to prevent mouth snapping down on cervix
* Allow blades to close naturally as you remove speculum and rotate handles horizontally to exit vagina
* Dispose of speculum and gloves.

Finishing off

- Thank patient
- Cover them up/ comfortable
- Offer patient tissue to wipe up
- Allow patient privacy to get dressed
- Wash hands.

Also:

- Warn patient they may experience some bleeding over the next few days
- Explain that the results will take 4–8 weeks to arrive via post
- Form notes:
  - Patient details
  - Reason for smear – routine
  - Pregnant/ menopausal
  - Currently using COCP/ HRT
  - Last menstrual period (LMP).

Common Paediatric Cases

Introduce yourself to the child and parent/carer, clarifying your role and task. Avoid asking permission from the child as they may refuse and hinder the rest of the station! Establish rapport and befriend the child by, for example, asking their name and age and get down to their level. This is essential for cooperation and in identifying clinical findings, but also shows the examiner that you are comfortable and well-rehearsed at examining children and infants.

In contrast to adults, the examination of children is opportunistic and it is important to preserve modesty. Undress and dress the child appropriately when asked to examine specific systems. It is often helpful to talk through your examination demonstrating to the examiner important positive and negative findings.

ACE TIPS

- Wash hands and introduce yourself

- Use informal observation at start

- Position and expose the child appropriately

- Be gentle and kind yet confident

- Do not cause pain or distress to child/parent

General

Position

- Babies can be examined on a couch or cot mattress
- Infants can be examined whilst on a parent's lap or over their shoulder. By keeping the child close to the parent you are less likely to upset them
- Preschool children can be examined whilst playing, for example.

Informal observation

This is the most useful and informative part of any paediatric examination and can provide you with important information:

- Is the child well or unwell?
- Is the child well-grown or malnourished?
- Is the child's behaviour normal or abnormal?
- Is this child's development normal or abnormal?
- Is this child dysmorphic or syndromic?

Asthma

General inspection/observation

- Bedside – oxygen, inhaler/nebuliser, spacers, peak flow device
- Inadequately controlled asthma – failure to thrive/ nutritional status?

- Other features of atopic disease – e.g., eczematous skin
- Cushingoid from long-term steroid use?
- Hyperinflated appearance of chest or pectus carinatum (pigeon chest)
- Harrison's sulci (indentation of the chest wall along the costal margins where the diaphragm inserts) – suggestive of chronic asthma.

ACE TIPS

- Ask to plot the child's height and weight on an appropriate growth chart

- Thank the child and parent/carer at the end of the examination

---

Palpation
- Usually symmetrical chest expansion (maybe reduced in chronic asthma).

Percussion
- Resonant unless complicated by pneumothorax or consolidation.

Auscultation
- Vesicular
- Wheeze?
- Beware of transmitted sounds, listen over the throat and compare it with the chest. If they are the same they are likely to be transmitted.

ACE TIPS

Asthma

- Family and social history

- Severity of asthma – missed school/sleep; admissions to hospital; past and present treatment; frequency of symptoms/reliever inhaler use

- Check inhaler technique

- Request to measure peak flow

- Parental education essential

Bronchiolitis

General inspection/observation
- Infant
- Wet, moist sounding cough
- Evidence of respiratory distress, i.e., recession, tracheal tug, tachypnoea (count the respiratory rate)

- Feeding supplementation, e.g., nasogastric tube
- Oxygen supplementation, e.g., nasal cannulae
- Intravenous infusion of fluids.

Palpation

- Liver displaced downwards.

Auscultation

- Fine, end-inspiratory crackles throughout the lung fields
- High-pitched wheezing.

Inflammatory bowel disease

General inspection

- Clubbing, leuconychia (hypoalbuminaemia)?
- Nutritional status – malnourished?
- Pallor?
- Nasogastric or gastrostomy feeding tube?
- Mouth ulcers?
- Skin – erythema nodosum, pyoderma gangrenosum
- Ask to inspect the anal and perianal region – fistulae, abscesses etc.

Palpation

- Scars
- Stoma (colostomy or ileostomy depending upon site of disease)
- Palpate all quadrants of the abdomen for tenderness
- Hepatomegaly if associated hepatobiliary disease, e.g., sclerosing cholangitis.

ACE TIPS

Inflammatory bowel disease

- Multidisciplinary management including dietetic input

- Plot height and weight on growth chart

- Various radiological investigations, e.g., barium meal

- Be aware of the mainstay of treatment e.g. steroids and immunomodulators etc.

- Pyscho-social impact on child and family

Cerebral palsy

General inspection/observation

- Wheelchair/reduced mobility?
- Visual impairment (squints/glasses etc)?

- Hearing aids?
- Shoe support?
- Tone and posturing?
- Feeding support, e.g., gastrostomy tube?
- Any deformity or scoliosis?
- Hemiplegia/ quadriplegia/ diplegia?
- Abnormal speech and language?

ACE TIPS

Cerebral palsy

- Revise aetiologies and types of cerebral palsy

- Multidisciplinary management

- Medical treatment including associated epilepsy

- Do not forget to assess gait if they can walk

- Special aids and education

- Pyscho-social impact on child and family

Cystic fibrosis
General inspection/observation
- Small – failure to thrive
- Scars from previous Hickman line insertion (long-term antibiotic use)
- Clubbed, cyanosed
- Halitosis
- Hyper-inflated, with Harrison's sulci
- Look in the sputum pot (purulent).

Palpation
- Reduced chest expansion.

Percussion
- Resonant unless there is consolidation.

Auscultation
- Wheeze
- Coarse crackles.

SPECIALITIES : 36. Common Paediatric Cases

ACE TIPS

Cystic fibrosis

- Autosomal recessive condition, present in 1/2500 births

- The gene, CFTR, encodes a protein which is a component of chloride channel

- Complications include chronic pancreatitis, infertility

- Management is multi-disciplinary

Down's syndrome (Trisomy 21)

General inspection
- Round face
- Epicanthic folds
- Flat occiput
- Squint
- Protruding tongue
- Brushfield spots in iris
- Slanted palpebral fissures
- Small ears
- Abnormal creases on palms and soles.

Palpation
- Hypotonia (posture/handling) especially in infants
- Third fontanelle.

ACE TIPS

Down's syndrome

- Know the background cytogenetics

- Commonest genetic cause of severe learning difficulty

- Be aware of the associations and later complications, e.g., thyroid disease

- Congenital heart disease (40%) and intestinal atresia are common

Nephrotic syndrome

General inspection/observation
- Periorbital oedema
- Oedema elsewhere e.g., scrotal, leg
- Commoner in boys.

Palpation
* Abdominal distension.

Percussion
* Ascites.

Auscultation
* Reduced breath sounds if pleural effusion.

ACE TIPS

Nephrotic symdrome

* Ask for blood pressure and urine dip analysis (heavy proteinuria)

* Usually steroid-responsive

* This is the triad of oedematous hypoalbuminaemia and protein in the urine

---

Eczema

General inspection
* Red/itchy/raised/excoriated lesions
* Distribution varies with age, e.g., infant – face; older child – flexor regions
* May be dry or weeping
* Symmetrical
* Does the child have any features of atopic disease, e.g. asthma?

ACE TIPS

Eczema

* Enquire about family history

* Conservative and medical management

* Be aware of the common precipitants/causes of exacerbations

* Majority of cases resolve by teenage years

Common causes of an itchy rash in an infant/child
1. Eczema
2. Chickenpox
3. Scabies
4. Allergic reactions/urticaria.

Neurocutaneous cases

Neurofibromatosis type 1

- Café-au-lait spots
- Autosomal dominant – family history
- Iris hamartomas (Lisch nodules)
- Axillary or inguinal freckling.

Other causes of café-au-lait patches

- Tuberous sclerosis
- Ataxia telangiectasia
- McCune–Albright syndrome
- Normal variant.

Tuberous sclerosis

- Adenoma sebaceum – fibrous angiomatous lesions in a butterfly distribution
- Hypopigmented "ash-leaf" patches (fluoresce under ultraviolet light)
- Shagreen patches – roughened areas usually over sacrum/lumbar spine
- Triad of epilepsy, mental retardation/intellectual impairment and developmental delay (with infantile spasms).

Sturge–Weber syndrome

- Facial port wine stain in the distribution of the trigeminal nerve (ophthalmic division always involved)
- Associated with similar intracranial lesion
- Associated with epilepsy, learning difficulties and contralateral hemiplegia.

⊙ Mental State Examination

The complexity to this examination stems from there being so many words to use to describe your patient. The art of the mental state examination is learning how to choose the best one.

Not only is the mental state examination explained here, but a list of the most helpful terms to use in trying to describe your findings has been provided.

Appearance
• State the patient's sex, ethnic origin, and age:
  – "The patient is a Caucasian man in his mid twenties."
• Comment on the dress:
  – Is the patient's dress appropriate to the weather?
  – Is the patient's dress appropriate to the circumstance or is it bizarre?
• Does the patient appear well kempt or unkempt?
  – Are the clothes dirty?
  – Is the patient unshaven with messy hair?
  – Is the patient malnourished thin due to self neglect?
• Are their any signs of self harm?
• If the interview is in the patients home or hospital room, inspect the appearance of surrounding environment.
  – "The patient's room was littered in cigarette butts and waste food."

Behaviour
• Are their any signs of self harm?
• Does the patient seem alert or confused?
• Does the patient seem calm or agitated?
• Any specific characteristics, e.g., are they withdrawn or tearful (takes practice!)?
• Does the patient's mental state appear to influence their movements? The patient who is fidgety, pacing up and the down room demonstrates psychomotor agitation. The motionless patient demonstrates psychomotor retardation.
• Always comment on whether you felt good rapport was established? Explain your reasons for your opinion:
  – Good rapport – the patient was cooperative and pleasant.
  – Poor rapport – the patient was hostile, guarded, indifferent, distracted or disinhibited.
• Always comment on whether the patient maintained good eye contact with you.
• Note any inappropriate conduct – did they swear at you/ were they aggressive?

Speech

- Assess the quality of the patient's speech:
    - Was their speech clear or slurred?
    - Volume – did they speak too quietly or did they shout?
- Rate:
    - Did you find that they could not be interrupted? (pressure of speech)
    - Did they seem hesitant to speak with a delay before starting? (poverty of speech)
- Assess the quantity of the patient's speech:
    - Did they speak too much or too little?
    - Did they speak spontaneously or only in response to your questions?

Mood

Make an objective assessment of the patient's mood, including:

- Inquire about the patient's mood (subjective assessment).
- Record what they say:
    - "I feel like so upset and annoyed doctor."

Affect

This is your observation of a patient's emotional state at a particular moment in time:

Useful terms to help describe a patient's mood
• Low in mood
• Euthymic
• Elated
• Anxious
• Angry
• Apathetic
• Agitated

- It is important to distinguish this term from the patient's mood.
- Follow this analogy – "It may be summer in season but raining this morning," i.e., someone may be euthymic in their mood but may be tearful in affect when talking about something sad.
- Assess the quality of the patient's speech.
- What triggers the patients affect to change during the interview?
    - "The patient's affect was within the normal range. When we spoke of the death of his father, he seemed sad, but when we spoke about his two children he seemed happy."

Three essential terms to grasp regarding affect are as follows:

- Blunted – the patient's face and body language show little emotion and their voice is monotonous.
- Flat – here there is even less emotional expression than seen with a blunted affect.
- Labile – the patient's emotional state fluctuates during a short period of time: one moment they are laughing, then the next they are crying, then again they are laughing.

Is the patient's affect congruent with the context of discussion? When talking about the death of a loved one, does the patient laugh? This is known as mood incongruency.

Risk assessment

- Always assess the patient's risk of suicide, homicide and self harm.
  - "Do you feel or have you been feeling that your life is not worth living?"
  - "Have you wanted to harm yourself or harm others?"

Thought form

There are a number of technical terms used to describe signs of abnormal thought form. They can be divided into two groups – those where you can identify a connection between the patient's thoughts and those where you can not.

- Connection between things said (bipolar)
  - Circumstantial – having asked a question of the patient, they seem to take forever to answer the question, digressing onto topics that you did not ask them about. Eventually, however, they do answer your question.
  - Tangential – having asked a question of the patient, they digress onto topics that you did not ask them about and fail to return to address your question.
  - Flight of ideas – the patient has racing thoughts and this manifests with pressure of speech. The connection between the patient's thoughts is seen through punning or clang association.
- No connection between things said (schizophrenia)
  - This is known as "loosening of associations" (or as formal thought disorder).
  - There are three types:
    1. Derailment
    2. Knight's move
    3. Word salad.

Other things to listen out for:

- Neologisms – makes up new words
- Perseveration – repeats one word recently said by themselves
- Echolalia – repeats words recently heard from others.

Thought content

There are three types of abnormal thought content:

- Abnormal beliefs/ delusions – these are false ideas that the patient continues to believe despite all attempts to convince them otherwise, and that are not shared by their culture or religion.
- Obsessions – these are false ideas that the patient believes are irrational but recurrently and spontaneously enter into the patients mind to cause them distress.
- Overvalued ideas – these are ideas that may not be false. They are not irrational to the patient. They dominate a patient's life:
  - "I am fat and I need to loose 10 pounds to be thin so I have been starving myself."

> **Definitions**
>
> • **Persecutory:** believes others are trying to harm them
>
> • **Grandiose:** believes they have special powers
>
> • **Reference:** believes things around them have a special meaning to themselves, such as the TV or radio is communicating directly to them
>
> • **Control (passivity):** believes their actions are controlled by an external force.
>
> • **Thought insertion/ withdrawal/ broadcasting:** believes someone/thing has put thoughts into their head, or has removed thoughts from their head or that others can read their mind
>
> • **Nihilistic:** believes their body is rotting
>
> • **Infestation:** believes their insects are crawling on their body
>
> • **Misidentification:** believes that their loved one has been replaced by an imposter

Abnormal perceptions

The most important type of abnormal perception is an hallucination. These are perceptions that happen in the absence of any external physical stimuli. They appear real to the patient and as if coming from outside their head.

• Auditory hallucinations are most common – the patient may hear voices echoing their thoughts, talking to them, or talking about them.

• Hallucinations may also be visual or tactile.

Cognition

• A full mini mental state examination should be performed and the result recorded.

Insight

If the patient does not believe they have a mental health problem, they are not going to want to have treatment. To assess likeliness of treatment compliance, assess their insight.

• "Do you think you have a (mental health) problem?"

• "What do you think is the cause of this problem?"

• "Do you think you need help for this problem?"

• "Would you like to have treatment for this problem?"

Insight may be graded as full insight, partial insight, or lacking insight.

Case presentation

Having completed your examination, summarize your findings. "This patient is a Caucasian man in his mid-twenties. He was bizarrely dressed, wearing bright orange shorts and a T-shirt that he had consciously cut into and sunglasses. He was, however, well kempt. Though he was alert, he seemed agitated. Good rapport was not established as he was disinhibited, asking provocative questions and at times swearing. He did maintain good eye contact. His speech appeared pressured. He seemed elated in mood, and he said he "felt on top of the world". His affect was within the normal range and he was mood congruent. He is not suicidal. He demonstrated flight of ideas and often used clang associations. He believed he has special powers that he was going to heal the world with the help of famous footballers. He had no abnormal perceptions. He was not oriented in time or place and was lacking insight into why he was in hospital."

Skin Lesion Examination

Summary

☐ Patient suitably exposed.

☐ State the site you are looking at.

☐ State the distribution of the skin lesion. Is it localized or generalized?

☐ Then assess whether the lesion is less than 0.5 cm or greater than 0.5 cm in size.

☐ Proceed to describe the characteristics of the lesion you have identified.

    ☐ Shape

    ☐ Edge

    ☐ Colour

☐ Look for secondary features and describe these using the terms given above.

☐ Summarise your findings and offer a diagnosis.

Examiner's instruction

"Here is an image of a patient with a skin lesion. Please describe what you observe and offer a diagnosis."

Wh Wash hands

I Introduce yourself and identify patient

S Summarise how you would like to examine the patient

P Permission

E Expose the patient suitably

R Reposition patient

S State of patient (well/unwell).

Stand at the end of the bed and look at the patient

> **ACE TIPS**
>
> Ask the patient if they are in any pain before you touch them

Site

"Here is an image of a man, and I am looking at his knees."

Distribution

Now state the distribution of any skin lesion. Distribution can be described as *localized* or *generalized*. If the lesion is localized, are you looking at one lesion or multiple skin lesions? Describe multiple lesions in a localized area as a *cluster*. Does the cluster follow a *linear* or *circular pattern*, or is it *curved (arcuate)*. Be aware of any obvious patterns of distribution:

• Peripheral vs. central

• Symmetrical vs. asymmetrical

• Flexors vs. extensors

• Sun exposed

• Dermatomal.

"There is a single localized symmetrical skin lesion present on the extensor aspect of both knees."

Size

Assess whether the lesion is less than or greater than 0.5 cm (can be 1 cm cut off). The words used to describe a lesion vary depending on the size (see Table).

"I would describe the skin lesion as a plaque as it is large and raised above the skin surface."

Characteristics

• Shape:

  • Circular, linear, nummular – looks like a coin

  • Annular – looks like a ring

  • If you can't describe any obvious shape, just say "irregular"

The lesion	<0.5 cm	0.5–2 cm	>2 cm
Flat with the skin	Macule	Patch	
Raised above skin	Papule	Nodule	Plaque
Fluid filled blister	Vesicle	Bulla	
Pus filled blister	Pustule	Abscess	
Oedema into skin	Wheal	Angioedema	
Extravasation of blood into skin	Petechia, purpura	Ecchymosis, haematoma	

[1]

- Edge:
  - A clear outline to the lesion makes it well marginated
  - A poor outline makes it ill defined
- Colour.

"The plaques are irregular in shape, well marginated and erythematous (red)."

Secondary features

The terms used to describe these features are specialized to dermatology, and will impress any examiner (see Box).

Secondary features

Crust: dried blood or pus

Scale: flaking skin

Pigmentation: lightening or darkening of the skin

Keratosis: raised thickening of the skin

Lichenification: thickening of skin with skin markings due to long term scratching

Erosion: area of epidermal loss

Excoriation: erosion caused by scratching

Fissure: linear split in epidermis

Ulcer: area of epidermal and dermal loss

"There is associated scaling of the lesion. The scaling is silvery."

Finishing off

- Thank the patient
- Make sure patient is comfortable and offer to help cover them up

- Wash hands
- Present and form differential
- Summarise.

Case presentation

"The image shows well-marginated plaques on the extensor aspect of the knees topped with silvery scale consistent with the findings in plaque psoriasis."

Interpreting a Chest X-ray

A chest X-ray (CXR) is an excellent station for medical final exams. It is a flexible station that can be used to assess not only the candidates X-ray knowledge, but also generic skills important to practising as a foundation year doctor. It is ideally suited to an OSCE station, both static and interactive.

The following skills can be assessed in a CXR OSCE station:

- Interpretive skills
- Communication skills – oral and written
- Structure and logic
- The ability to construct a differential diagnosis
- Clinical correlation
- Decision-making skills.

Although a range of X-rays could be chosen as an OSCE station a chest X-ray is by far the most likely as:

- It is the commonest X-ray investigation requested.
- It can be vital to out-of-hours management decisions.
- It is a fair investigation to expect a foundation doctor to interpret.

The key points to bear in mind in a CXR OSCE are:

- Don't be scared.
- Know the anatomy of a CXR.
- Approach it systematically.
- Describe what you see and the diagnosis will follow.
- Avoid getting tangled with using too many words.
- Give a confident summary to end.

Systematic approach to chest X-ray interpretation

Although individuals will approach a CXR in various ways, a suggested systematic approach is shown here for reference. Practice with colleagues and you will soon become more comfortable, just as with a clinical systems examination.

- Film specifics (name, age, DOB, ward, patient's consultant)
- Technical factors (film projection, rotation, inspiration, penetration)
- Heart and major vessels
- Lungs and pleura
- Mediastinum (including hila)
- Bones
- Soft tissues.

Anatomy of a normal chest X-ray

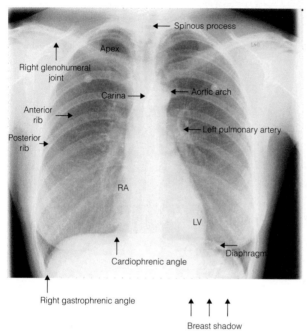

Normal chest X-ray

Review areas:

The review areas should be specifically checked as abnormalities in these areas are easily overlooked. These are:

- Apices
- Behind the heart
- Below the diaphragms
- The hila
- Breast shadows (in females).

Complete your assessment

Provide the following:

- A 3–4 line summary
- A differential diagnosis list with . . .
- The most likely (your impression) first.

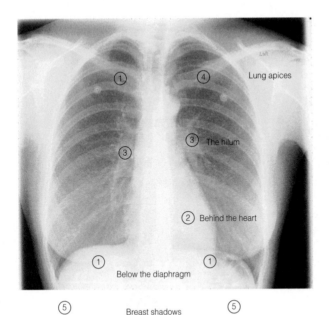

The review areas:

1. Below the diaphragm

2. Behind the heart

3. The hilum

4. Lung apices

5. Breast shadows

ACE TIPS

- A chest X-ray (CXR) is the most likely X-ray in final exams.

- Don't forget a CXR is a two-dimensional representation of three-dimensional structures.

- Satisfaction of search – don't be content with finding one abnormality, keep looking for more. It may hold the key to the definitive diagnosis.

- An anteroposterior (AP) projection magnifies the heart so don't comment on heart size.

- Remember the review areas – forget at your peril.

- Be succinct with your report – make every word count.

Common OCSE cases

- Cardiac failure
- Pleural effusion
- Pneumothorax
- Bronchial carcinoma
- Lobar pneumonia or collapse

Examiner's instruction

"Please read the following clinical vignette then assess and interpret the patient's chest X-ray."

Example chest X-ray station

This 72-year-old lady attended hospital short of breath (Mrs Z Ljubljana, DOB 12-08-1935). She is a smoker of 40 pack years.

On examination: tar staining; grade 2 finger clubbing; respiratory examination unremarkable.

Please assess the patient's CXR, giving a differential diagnosis.

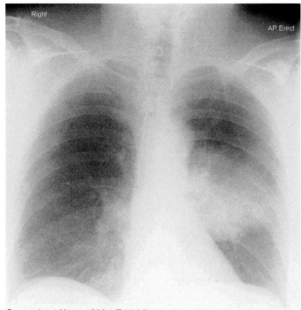

Case: chest X-ray of Mrs Z Ljubljana

Case presentation

Chest X-ray report

AP erect chest X-ray

Mrs Z Ljubljana, 72-year-old lady, DOB 12-08-1935.

The technical quality of the film is satisfactory.

7 cm mass in the left mid zone, centred on the left hilum. No adjacent rib destruction. The right lung is normal.

The differential diagnosis includes bronchial carcinoma, pulmonary metastasis, round pneumonia and lung abscess.

Examiner's questions:

1. What is the most likely cause?

   Bronchial carcinoma

2. What further investigations would be of help?

   Staging CT of chest and abdomen; bronchoscopy

3. How is this condition classified histologically?

   Small cell and non-small cell lung cancer. Non-small cell includes squamous cell carcinoma, adenocarcinoma and large cell lung cancer.

Doctor details: Dr T Simpson, FY1 doctor, Bleep 008

Signature: *Dr T Simpson*   **Date:** 29/09/07

⚫ Interpreting an Abdominal X-ray

An abdominal X-ray (AXR) is a fair station for medical final exams. It is likely to feature in a surgical type scenario, as it is in these patients where it has its greatest utility. The chief indications for an AXR are for bowel obstruction, including toxic megacolon, and in suspected renal colic. It should be requested sparingly given the risk:benefit ratio of providing a diagnosis against its dose – 35 times that of a CXR. One should be particularly thoughtful in women of child-bearing age. Alternative imaging investigations, particularly ultrasound, are often more helpful.

The following skills can be assessed in an AXR OSCE station:

- Interpretive skills
- Communication skills – oral and written
- Structure and logic
- The ability to construct a differential diagnosis
- Clinical correlation
- Decision-making skills.

Although a range of X-rays could be chosen as an OSCE station, an abdominal X-ray is one of the most likely as:

- It is the second commonest plain X-ray that foundation years will review alone out of hours.
- It can be vital to out-of-hours management decisions, especially in surgical patients.
- It is a fair investigation to expect a foundation doctor to interpret.
- Is frequently accompanied with an erect CXR for a "surgical abdomen" patient.

The key points to bear in mind in an AXR OSCE are:

- Don't be scared.
- Know the anatomy of the AXR.
- Be aware of its limitations in making a diagnosis.
- Approach it systematically.
- Describe what you observe and the diagnosis will follow.
- Avoid getting tangled with using too many words.
- Give a confident summary to end.
- Request sparingly as the dose is 35 times that of a CXR.

Systematic approach to abdominal X-ray interpretation

Although individuals will approach an AXR in various ways, a suggested systematic approach is shown here for reference. Practice with colleagues and you will soon become more comfortable, just as with a clinical systems examination.

- Film specifics
- Technical factors (is the whole abdomen covered and of adequate penetration)
- Bowel calibre and distribution

- Soft tissues
- Bones
- Any abnormal calcific densities (e.g., a renal calculus) or artefact (e.g., sterilisation clips) on the film.

Anatomy of a normal abdominal X-ray

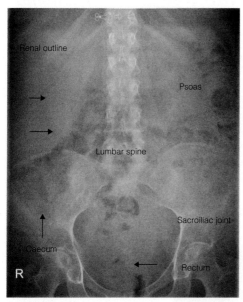

Normal abdominal X-ray

Complete your assessment

Provide the following:

- A 3–4 line summary
- A differential diagnosis list:
  - The most likely (your impression) first.

ACE TIPS

- An AXR is not the plain film of choice for a clinical suspicion of pneumoperitoneum, it is an erect CXR.

- Check the hernial orifices with bowel obstruction. A hernia may be the cause.

- Air on either side of the bowel wall or triangular areas of gas indicate pneumoperitoneum

- Renal calculi are identified much more frequently than gallstones.

Common OSCE cases

- Small bowel obstruction
- Large bowel obstruction
- Toxic megacolon
- Renal calculus
- Pneumoperitoneum

Examiner's instruction

"Please read the following clinical vignette then assess and interpret the patient's abdominal X-ray."

Example abdominal X-ray station

This 74-year-old lady attended hospital with a distended abdomen and vomiting. (Mrs L Bled, DOB 15-02-1933). Her previous history includes a hysterectomy.

On examination: distended abdomen; reduced bowel sounds.

Please assess the patient's AXR, including your clinicoradiological impression.

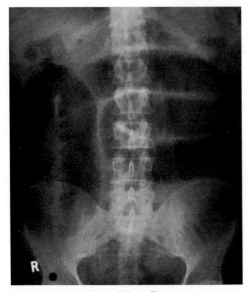

Case: abdominal X-ray of Mrs L Bled

Case presentation

Abdominal X-ray report

Abdominal X-ray

Mrs L Bled, 74-year-old lady, DOB 15-02-1933.

The technical quality of the film is satisfactory.

Multiple loops of distended small bowel, measuring approximately 4cm, within the central abdomen. Paucity of gas within the large bowel. No groin hernias.

Findings consistent with small bowel obstruction.

Answers to examiner's questions:

1. What is the most likely diagnosis?

   Small bowel obstruction

2. What are the causes of this condition, and which is the most likely in this case?

   The commonest cause is surgical adhesions, as is likely in this case given the history of a hysterectomy. Other causes include: hernia, volvulus and an intraluminal mass such as a small bowel lymphoma.

3. What further imaging investigation may be of help?

   CT of the abdomen. Depending on the patient's status, clinical preferences and institution further imaging may be performed.

Doctor details: Dr S Kitson, FY1 doctor, Bleep 008

Signature: *Dr S Kitson*   **Date:** 30/09/07

Medical Statistics

Ever wondered why we treat patients the way we do? In the era of modern medicine, it is all about evidence-based medicine. Gone are the days of unregulated professionals and quacks providing new and radical treatments. Evidence-based medicine is the continuous search and modification of practice so as to gain the best evidence in making decisions about the care of individual patients.

Due to its implications and significance, it is important for students to understand the basic concepts of medical statistics and how to appraise the hundreds of studies conducted in the field, before graduation. As such, it forms an integral part of OSCE examinations in finals.

Basic terminology

Mean: the average value:

$$\frac{a+b+c+d+e}{5}$$

Mode: the most frequent value in a sequence:

$$a, a, b, b, b, b, c, d, e = b$$

Median: the middle number when values placed numerically:

$$a, b, c, d, e, f, g = d$$

$$\text{Incidence} = \frac{\text{number of } new \text{ cases}}{\text{population}}$$

$$\text{Prevalence} = \frac{\text{number of } existing \text{ cases}}{\text{population}}$$

$$\text{Mortality} = \frac{\text{number of deaths}}{\text{population}}$$

Diagnostic testing and screening

A diagnostic test is a tool used to detect a disease. Screening is a method of establishing the presence of a condition before it has developed or in its early stages. Screening is a great concept as it allows the clinician to identify and potentially treat a condition early on. There are many criteria that a screening process must fulfil. It must be a significant disease with an established and an effective treatment regimen for the majority of cases. The tool must be as non-invasive as possible (and ideally must be something that you would be willing to have done to yourself). Current well-established screening programmes include mammography for breast cancer. New ones on the horizon could be prostate serum antigen (PSA) screening for prostatic cancer or ultrasonography for abdominal aortic aneurysms.

Criteria for a screening programme

- Significant disease

- Existence of an effective treatment regimen

- Valid test

- Cost effective

- Quick and as noninvasive as possible

- Acceptable to the population

Once a screening tool is in practice, its effectiveness needs to be investigated. This is done by looking at its sensitivity, specificity and predictive values:

- **Sensitivity:** percentage of truly diseased people who are identified as diseased by the test under study

- **Specificity:** percentage of truly non-diseased patients who are identified as non-diseased by the test under study

- **Predictive value:** probability that a person with a positive/negative test is truly positive/negative.

	Disease +ve	Disease −ve	
Test +ve	a	b	a + b
Test +ve	c	d	c + d
Total	a + c	b + d	

Sensitivity = a/(a + c)
Specificity = d/(b + d)
+ve PV = a/(a + b)
−ve PV = c/(c + d)

Trials

Clinical trials are important in medical practice. They have many uses. They provide an effective way of comparing and contrasting different drug or treatment regimens against one another. They can also be used to look at the history of progression or potential causative factors in a condition. There are many types of studies, however, we will focus only on the three main types: randomised controlled studies, case control studies and cohort studies.

Some types of studies

- Interventional aka randomised controlled trials (RCT)

- Case-control studies

- Cohort studies

- Systematic reviews

- Ecological studies

- Cross-sectional studies

(Randomised) controlled studies

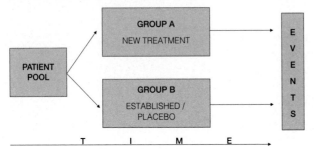

Randomised controlled studies

In this type of study there are two groups. One group which receives the treatment under investigation (treatment group) and another group which receives either no treatment (placebo) or an already established or standard treatment (control group).

Randomisation is a process of randomly allocating patients to each group so as to try and achieve maximal similarity between the two groups.

These can be expensive and time consuming to conduct and a question of ethics may arise – is it ethical to deprive some patients of a potentially new and therapeutic drug? Or, conversely, is it safe to subject patients to new drugs (e.g., Northwick Park trial)?

Randomised controlled trials

Advantages:

• Blinded – single/double

• Randomisation

• Compare between established treatments or placebo

Disadvantages:

• Expensive

• Time consuming

• Confounding factors

• Bias

• Ethical?

• Not useful for rare disease

Case-control studies

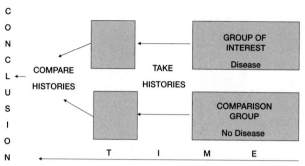

Case control studies

In this type of study, we compare a group of patients who already have a certain condition against a similar group of patients who do not have it.

It does not involve recruiting patients and can be done via questionnaires, patient notes or direct contact with patients. This can also be a disadvantage as patients may not recall exactly the questions being asked and so results could potentially be misleading. Also confounding may play a significant role.

Case-control studies

Advantages:

- Good for conditions with long latencies

- Good for rare disease

- Easy to "recruit"

- Quick

- Cheap

- Potential to look at multiple factors

Disadvantages:

- Recall bias

- Confounding factors

- Relationship may or may be true

- Choice of comparison group may be difficult

Cohort studies

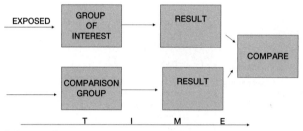

Cohort studies

In this type of study, one group of patients who have a certain disease (and may receive a particular treatment) are compared against a similar group not affected by that condition. The different outcomes are followed over time to see what health problems may develop.

Cohort studies

Advantages:

* Reduces bias

* Potential to look at multiple factors

Disadvantages:

* Time consuming

* Confounding factors

* Relationship may or may be true

* Choice of comparison group may be difficult

* Loss to follow-up

* Exposure pattern can change over time

* Not useful for rare disease

Other types of studies

Systematic reviews: this is not strictly speaking a study. It is a literature review whereby lots of similar studies are reviewed and all the results pooled together to try and come to a more precise and accurate conclusion. They can be very accurate but are prone to some problems. Not all studies conducted around a similar study are comparable and this leads to the problem of *comparability*. Another issue that needs to be considered is *publication bias*. Are all studies conducted published and reviewed? Are studies conducted in different countries or published in different languages considered?

Ecological studies: in this type of study, the unit of comparison is a population or community. Disease rates and exposures are measured and compared against other populations or communities. It is relatively easy and cheap to conduct. The main problem is that of ecological fallacy. This draws a presumptive assumption that all members of the group exhibit, largely, the same characteristics.

Interpreting the numbers

Every study needs to come to a conclusion, whether positive or negative. The way that the figures are presented can be misleading though, and readers should be able to understand and make a decision for themselves as to the significance or not of the conclusions drawn by the authors. Remember, if the investigators have poured a lot of money and time into a study, they may not be too keen to dismiss the findings, and so present the data in such a way as to justify their claims.

Relative risk (RR)

How many times more likely exposed persons are to get the disease compared with those who are unexposed.

Odds ratio (OR)

Equivalent of an RR in a case-control study.

Disease	Yes	No
Exposed	a	b
Unexposed	c	d

$$RR = \frac{a/(a+b)}{c/(c+d)}$$

$$OR = ad/bc$$

Number needed to treat

Number of patients needed to treat in order to improve the outcome of a *single* patient.

This is 1/absolute risk reduction.

p value

This value predicts how likely the relationship under investigation is due to chance. It is important to understand that the lower the p value, the more likely that a true relationship exists between the factors under investigation. Thus a p value of <0.005 means there is less than 0.1% chance that the relationship under investigation is due to chance; it is therefore statistically significant, and so a potential risk association may exist.

95% confidence interval

This is a statistical range of numerical values between which we can be 95% sure that the population value under investigation exists; i.e., we are 95% sure that the true test result lies between these two values. The importance in this value is looking at how wide this interval is and whether or not it crosses 1. Confidence intervals indicate the strength of the findings. The narrower the interval the more precise the evidence is. A larger study will tend to have a narrower interval than a smaller one. The other important implication of this interval is whether or not it crosses 1. If it does, it means that the exposure could have either a beneficial or detrimental effect and thus is statistically insignificant. This would call for further investigation of the potential relationship. For example:

95% CI: 0.78–1.43 = Insignificant

95% CI: 0.78–0.87 = Significant

95% CI: 3.65–7.82 = Significant

Bias

This is a problem in conducting trials and measures are in place to try and minimise bias. Bias occurs when factors/people cause skewing of results in one direction or another; for example, researchers may try and shed more of a positive light on a new drug. This can be eliminated by blinding of the trial.

- **Measurement or recall bias** refers to inaccuracies in subjects recalling precisely how much exposure they had to the stimulus under investigation; e.g., asking people how long they speak on their mobile phones a day.

- **Selection bias** refers to favouring either the control or treatment group in order to try and skew the results in either direction. This can be eliminated by randomisation.

Confounding factors

These are factors outside our search criteria that may or may not affect our results e.g., the association of miners and lung cancer but not including whether or not the subjects smoke as well. This can be partially solved by standardisation.

Blinding

This is a way of improving the validity of a study.

- In an **open study** both patient groups and researchers/clinicians know what treatment every patient is receiving. This could be a potential problem leading to measurement bias.

- **Single blinding** is when only one party (patients or researchers/clinicians) know what treatment they are receiving.

- **Double blinding** is the gold standard. Here neither party is aware of what treatment is being given.

Summary

Evidence-based medicine represents the core of modern day medical practice. It is essential to be able to understand all the terms and numbers put forward in the numerous medical journals that exist.

By understanding the basic concepts, one can make easy judgments and, importantly, pass the OSCE station easily.

ACE TIP

Remember: just because one study does or does not prove a statistically significant relationship does not mean that the relationship is true. More investigations should be done to support or dismiss the findings.

Example

Note: the case below is entirely fictional.

Examiner's instruction

"Please read the following extract and answer the questions below."

Incidence of testicular cancer in males and the carrying of mobile phones in trouser pockets, by Dr X in "The Journal of Made-Up Trials"

- **Aim:** to investigate the incidence of testicular cancer in males who carry mobile phones in their trouser pockets.

- **Methods:** case-control study in which 100 men of any age were chosen randomly from a GP database, fifty of whom did not own a mobile phone and fifty who did and carried it in any of their trouser pockets. Questionnaires with the following questions were sent:
  - Did they own a phone?
  - What make?
  - Type of fabric of trousers they wear?

- **Results:** of the fifty who did have a mobile phone, 11 developed testicular cancer. Only 2 of those who did not own a mobile phone developed cancer (OR 1.33, 95% CI: 1.02–1.67, p value 0.01).

- **Conclusion:** carrying a mobile phone in any trouser pocket significantly increases the risk of developing testicular cancer.

Questions and answers

1. What is a case-control study?

See text.

2. What was the aim of this study?

To look at the incidence of testicular cancer in males who carry a mobile phone in any of their pockets.

3. List three advantages and three disadvantages of this type of study?

See text.

4. Any potential problems in the recruitment and evaluation process?

Although they randomly selected patients from a GP database, they selected patients of any age and maybe should have focused on younger patients where the incidence of cancer is higher. Also, the questionnaire did not take into account family history or which pocket the phone was kept in (lower incidence in back pocket?).

5. Discuss the results.

The odds ratio supports a hypothesis that there is an increased risk of cancer in the study group. The 95% CI does not cross 1 and can therefore be seen to be statistically significant. The p value is not less than 0.005 suggesting that maybe there is no true relationship

6. Do you agree with the conclusion reached?

Bearing in mind the inadequacy of the questionnaire, possible unsuitability of the subjects and conflicting statistically results, no conclusions can be definitively drawn on any true association. This does not mean that here is no association between the two but further investigation will be necessary to determine this precisely.

7. What could be done to improve this trial?

More careful choice of subjects and a more detailed questionnaire.

Section IV
Practical Procedures

Inserting a Cannula

Examiner's instruction

"This model arm represents a man requiring cannualtion. He requires cannualtion for the commencement of IV antibiotics. Cannulate the model arm and communicate to the examiner as if they were the patient."

Wh Wash your hands

I Introduce yourself and identify patient (use their ID bracelet)

S Summarise how you would like to take blood from their arm why you need to put a catheter into their arm/hand

P Permission:

"Hello, my name is ... and I am a final year medical student. Can I just check your name please and your hospital number on your ID bracelet? I would like to insert a cannula, a plastic tube, into your arm by putting a needle covered by the plastic into your vein and quickly removing the needle so fluids and medicines can be given through the plastic without you having any more needles. You may feel a sharp scratch. Is that ok? Do you have any questions?"

E Equipment:
- Clean tray
- Pair of gloves
- Tourniquet
- Alcohol steret
- Gauze
- Sterile cap
- Cannula – pink or green
  - Blue for small veins
  - Grey for urgent resuscitation
- Cannula dressing
- Needle
- 5 ml sodium chloride 0.9% flush check it is in date
- 10 ml syringe.

R Reposition patient

S State of patient.

Procedure

- Put on gloves.
- Prepare the equipment for the flush.
- Confirm the name of the flush solution and the expiry date with an appropriate member of staff.
- Draw up at least 5 ml of solution into your syringe.
- Remove any excess air from the syringe.
- Carefully dispose of the needle into the sharps box.
- Replace the syringe into the packet.
- Prepare the sterile cap and cannula.
- Return to the patient.
- Apply the tourniquet and find a suitable vein.
- Clean the skin using the alcohol steret.
- Warn the patient of a sharp scratch.
- Insert the cannula into the vain at a 30-degree angle and watch for a flashback.
- Keeping the needle holder steady, insert the cannula plastic into the vein.
- Place gauze under the cannula to catch any spilled blood.
- Remove the tourniquet.
- Apply pressure over the vein to minimise blood spillage and withdraw the needle.
- Immediately place the needle into the sharps box.
- Screw in the flush syringe into the cap and introduce the flush.
- Screw in the sterile cap.
- Remove the gauze and apply the cannula dressing.

Finishing off

- Thank patient and make them comfortable.
- Remove your gloves and wash your hands.

Arterial Blood Gas

Wh Wash hands

I Introduce yourself and identify patient

S Summarise how you would like to take a blood sample from the artery in their wrist

P Permission

E Expose the arm, i.e., roll up the sleeve

E Equipment:
- Alcohol wipes
- Pre-heparinised syringe (3–5 ml) and 23 gauge needle
- Nonsterile gloves
- Gauze

R Reposition the arm flat

S State of patient.

Procedure

- Inspect the skin over the radial artery for cellulites.
- Extend the patient's wrist.
- Perform the Allen's test to check the collateral ulnar artery:
  - Rest the patients hand in their lap and compress both ulnar and radial artery simultaneously
  - Hold for 2 minutes whilst blood drains out of the hand
  - Release ulnar artery – if colour returns within 5–15 seconds, the test is positive as you can continue.
- Wear gloves.
- Locate radial artery.
- Cleanse site with alcohol swab – single stroke from centre outwards.
- Use a pre-heparinised syringe now.
- Attach new needle to syringe.
- Find radial artery and fix using tips of the fingers on either side.
- Warn the patient of a "sharp scratch".
- Insert needle at a 30 degree angle with needle bevel upwards.
- Guide needle towards pulsation.
- Once you puncture the artery, there is a flashback of arterial blood.
- Draw up 1–2 ml.
- Remove and discard the needle into the sharps bin.
- Expel any excess air in the syringe and cap it.

Finishing off

- Label specimen and say you would immediately process blood at an arterial blood gas (ABG) machine, accounting for the patient's oxygen requirements and temperature.
- Thank the patient
- Wash your hands.

● Venepuncture

Examiner's instruction

"This model arm represents a man requiring venepuncture, his name is Mr Tyler Foxton. Take a full blood count from the model arm and communicate to the examiner as if they were the patient."

ACE TIPS

- Ensure you identify you have the correct patient even when being asked to cannulate a model arm.

- Ensure you choose the correct blood bottle if specifically asked to collect blood for a specific test.

- Ensure you show the principles of identifying a vein even on the model arm.

- Do not leave the tourniquet on for too long during the procedure.

Wh Wash hands using the 7 stage technique

I   Introduce yourself and identify patient (use their ID bracelet)

S   Summarise how you would like to take blood from their arm and ask the patient if they have any questions

P   Permission – gain verbal consent.

"Hello, my name is . . . and I am a medical student. Can I just check your name please and your hospital number on your ID bracelet? I would like to take a sample of blood by quickly putting a needle into a vein so I can check that you have enough of all the important things in your blood. I have been asked to take a sample of your blood to check for . . . You may feel a sharp scratch. Is that OK?"

E   Equipment
- Clean tray
- Pair of gloves
- Tourniquet
- Alcohol steret
- Gauze
- Vacutainer barrel and needle (or needle and syringe)
- Blood bottles (as directed on the blood form or notes).

R   Reposition arm

S   State of patient.

Procedure
- Put on gloves.
- Attach the vacutainer needle to the barrel.
- Apply the tourniquet two fingers above the antecubital fossa.
- Find a suitable vein through sight and touch.
- Cleanse the skin using an alcohol steret.
- Remove the cap from the needle and warn the patient of a "sharp scratch".
- Hold the skin taut and insert the needle at 45 degrees into the vein and introduce the vacutainer blood bottle.
- Allow the blood to collect.
- Remove tourniquet and then the vacutainer bottle.
- Remove the needle from arm and safely dispose of the needle into the sharps bin.
- Apply cotton wool gauze to puncture site for 1 minute.

Finishing off
- Thank the patient and make them comfortable.
- Take off gloves.
- Wash hands.
- Label the blood bottle with:
  - Patients name
  - Date of collection
  - Ward
  - Time and date
  - Hospital number
  - Your signature.
- Label the blood form as appropriate.
- Seal the bottle in the blood form.

● Setting Up a Drip

Examiner's instruction

"You have been asked to set up an IV infusion as prescribed on Mr Tyler Night. Set up the IV infusion as prescribed, correctly attach to the cannula in the model arm and document."

ACE TIPS

• This station is often joined with the skill cannualtion.

• Ensure you identify you have the correct patient even when being asked to cannulate a model arm.

• Ensure prior to running through the drip you put the clamp on to minimise bubbles.

• Hospital policy in some places states that the IV infusion set should be attached via a bionectar connection not through a cannula port.

Wh Wash hands

I Introduce yourself and identify patient (use their ID bracelet)

S Summarise how you would like to set up a drip and ask if patient has any questions

P Permission – gain verbal consent:

"Hello my name is . . . I am a medical student. I would like to give you some fluids by passing them through the tube in your arm. Is that OK?"

E Expose the cannula, i.e., roll up the sleeve

E Equipment:
  • Nonsterile gloves
  • Fluid bag
  • Drip stand
  • Giving set
  • Connecting tube
  • 5 ml sodium chloride 0.9% flush; check it is in date
  • 10 ml syringe
  • Alcohol steret

R Reposition the arm flat

S State of patient.

Checks

• Check the drug chart to confirm:
  – the patients name, hospital no., D.O.B
  – the fluid prescription

- Check the fluid chart to monitor input and output
- Check the fluid bag to confirm:
  - The contents
  - Expiry date
- Ask a doctor or the examiner to cross check these details.

Procedure

- Put on non sterile gloves
- Draw up the sodium chloride flush into the syringe; if using a needle to do this dispose of the needle in a sharps bin and put the syringe back into the packaging.
- Inspect and clean cannula with steret and administer flush to check the cannula in situ for inflammation/extravasation.
- Ask if there is any pain where cannula is situated.
- Remove the fluid bag from the sterile packaging and hook it onto a drip stand inverted.
- Twist off the cap from the end of the fluid bag.
- Remove the giving set from sterile packaging and unwind the giving set.
- Close the valve on the giving set.
- Remove the cover from the giving set.
- Push the sharp end of the giving set into the bag outlet.
- Squeeze the drip chamber of the giving set till it is half full.
- Slowly open the valve to run the fluid to the end of the giving set tubing taking care not to trap air bubbles.
- In the presence of air bubbles briskly straighten the tube.
- Close the valve to prevent any spilled fluid.
- Remove the connecting tubing from the packet and connect it to the end of the giving set.
- Re-open the valve and ensure fluid flow.
- Insert the connect tubing into the cannula.
- Adjust the valve to set the drip rate.

Finishing off

- Sign the drug chart confirming that the fluid has been administered.
- Thank the patient.
- Dispose of gloves and wash your hands.

⊙ Intravenous Drug Administration

Examiner's instruction

"Mr Adam Day has been admitted for IV antibiotics. Draw up and deliver the drugs as prescribed via the cannula in the model arm. Document the giving of the medication."

> ### *ACE TIPS*
>
> * Ensure you identify that you have the correct patient even when being asked to cannulate a model arm.
>
> * Be aware that you shouldn't vigorously shake all drugs to disperse the diluent.
>
> * Ensure you read the prescription chart properly and document the delivery of the drug accurately after administration.

Wh Wash hands

I Introduce yourself and identify patient (use their ID bracelet)

S Summarise that you would like to give them IV antibiotics into their cannula

P Permission – gain verbal consent:

"Hello, my name is . . . and I am a medical student. Can I just check your name please and your hospital number and date of birth on your ID bracelet? I would like to give you some IV antibiotics to help you get better by passing it through the tube in your arm. Is that OK? Do you have any questions?"

E Equipment – for administration of a powder antibiotic that needs reconstituting:

* Clean tray
* Needles × 3
* Alcohol steret
* 5 ml bottle of 0.9% sodium chloride solution
* 5 ml bottle of solution for reconstitution or solution advised for reconstitution
* 10 ml syringe
* 5 ml syringe
* Medication as prescribed

R Reposition arm

S State of patient.

Safety check

* Ask the patient if they are allergic to the medication and confirm this from the drug chart.
* Confirm the prescription against the drug chart and against the drug vial.
* Check the drug has not just been given.
* Use the drug formulary sheets provided or the BNF for the volume of required diluent and the rate at which it should be administered.

Procedure

- Put on some gloves.
- Confirm the name of all medications and solutions, as well as the expiry dates with an appropriate member of staff.
- Remove the cap from the drug vial and clean it with a steret.
- Draw up the required volume of distilled water dilute in the syringe using a needle.
- Dispose of the needle into the sharps box.
- Draw up 5 ml of 0.9% sodium chloride solution for a flush and replace into packaging.
- Insert a fresh needle onto the syringe containing the distilled water.
- Inject all of the distilled water into the drug ampoule and shake until dispersed.
- Aspirate the dissolved solution back into the syringe and dispose of the needle into the sharps box.
- Return to the patient.
- Inspect the cannula for signs of infection and clean the end using a steret.
- Administer the medicine slowly at a rate directed by the drug formulary sheet or over a period of 2–3 minutes.

Patient warning

Observe the patient for signs of anaphylaxis:

- Stridor
- Wheeze + shortness of breath
- pale, cold, clammy, dizziness
- Loss of consciousness
- Rash.

Warn the patient that if they start to feel unwell in anyway they should let the nearest member of staff know

Finishing off

- Thank the patient and ensure they are comfortable.
- Wash your hands.
- Sign the drug chart.
- Cross sign the chart with an appropriate member of staff.

Hyperkalaemia Management

Examiner's instruction

"A 64 year old woman with a history of chronic kidney disease is admitted for treatment of a lower respiratory tract infection. Results of her U&E are phoned to you from the laboratory (see box). Describe what actions you would take to manage this patients hyperkalaemia."

U&E results	
Na^+	135 mmol/l
K^+	8.3 mmol/l
Cl^-	103 mmol/l
HCO_3^-	17 mmol/l
Urea	36 mmol/l
Creatinine	546 µmol/l
*Not haemolysed	

Hyperkalaemia is a medical emergency and can be life-threatening especially in patients with hyperkalaemia-induced electrocardiogram (ECG) changes. All foundation scheme doctors should know how to manage such an electrolyte emergency. Typically, the management of hyperkalaemia may appear as a modified essay question in medical finals. It may also take the form of an OSCE station, where you maybe assessed on your ability to prepare insulin therapy for the management of life-threatening hyperkalaemia. Incorrect administration of insulin therapy can cause serious patient harm, even death, so you should approach this problem carefully and with a systematic approach. It should be noted that, depending on the hospital, there may be different guidelines and you should always adhere to them.

Wh Wash hands

I Introduce yourself and identify the patient – it is good practice to verbally check the patients details and also check their identification bracelet

S Summarise to the patient what you are about to do

P Permission – gain the patients permission

E Exposure of patient – expose the patient's chest as you may be performing an ECG

R Reposition – ideally position the patient in a semirecumbent position

S State of patient – as in any procedure, it is always important to perform an appropriate clinical assessment of the patient.

Perform an electrocardiogram
You should initially request that an ECG should be performed. If this demonstrates features consistent with hyperkalaemia, you should decide that the patient requires treatment for this.

ECG features that are consistent with hyperkalaemia

These include:

• broad QRS complexes

• loss of P wave

• peaked T waves

Stabilization of the myocardium

If the ECG demonstrates features consistent with hyperkalaemia, consider administering 10 ml of 10% calcium gluconate IV to stabilise the patient's myocardium.

Preparation of insulin therapy

Now consider administering insulin therapy. Take the following steps:

• Put on a pair of gloves.

• You may suggest that you would like a second person to double check the preparation of the insulin therapy.

• Select 50 ml of 50% dextrose for infusion.

• Check the expiry date of the dextrose solution.

• Select actrapid insulin.*

• Check the expiry date of the insulin.

• Wipe the top of the insulin vial with an alcohol wipe.

• Select correct insulin syringe.*

• Draw up 5–10 UNITS of actrapid insulin with the insulin syringe.*

• Inject the insulin into the dextrose solution.

• Gently shake the combined mixture.

• Appropriately dispose of sharps and all other clinical waste.

• Prepare the solution for infusion by attaching a giving set.

These are critical steps and any errors here may result in an automatic fail.

Infusion of the dextrose/insulin solution

You may be asked to connect the dextrose/insulin solution and giving set to a cannula on a mannequin arm. If this is the case make sure to:

• Verbally check the patients identity and also check their identification bracelet.

• Inspect the cannula site.

• Swab the drug portal site of the cannula with an alcohol wipe.

• Administer a short flush of normal saline into the cannula.

• Connect the giving set and dextrose/insulin solution.

• Consider attaching a drip counter that will control the rate of infusion.

• Infuse the dextrose/insulin solution over at least 15 minutes.

• Keep the patient under close observation.

Monitoring

Following the administration of the dextrose/insulin solution you should:

* Monitor the clinical state of the patient
* Regular capillary blood glucose levels
* Repeat a U&E to ensure the K^+ level has reduced.

ACE TIPS

There are a number of potential measures that you can take to augment the effect of treatment of this electrolyte abnormality, including:

* Administer an inhaled β_2 agonist

* Stop any K^+ sparing medications

* Administer calcium resonium

* Renal dialysis

Finishing off

* Make a record of what you have done in both the patient's drug chart and medical notes.
* Thank the patient and ensure they are comfortable.
* Wash your hands.

Intramuscular Injection

Exam Instruction

"Miss Tina Yellow requires a tetanus booster after being bitten by her pet rabbit. Draw up the medication as prescribed and deliver the medication via the injection pad on the patients arm. Document the procedure."

ACE TIPS

- Ensure for an IM injection that the patient's skin is pulled taut prior to giving the injection

- Be aware of the signs of anaphylaxis

Wh Wash hands

I Introduce yourself and identify patient (use their ID bracelet)

S Summarise the procedure to patient and ask if they have any questions

P Permission – gain verbal consent

E Expose the injection site

E Equipment:
- Patient's drug chart
- Medication to be injected
- 10 ml syringe of appropriate size
- 21–23G gauge (blue or green) needle for injection
- 21G (green) needle for drawing up medication
- Alcohol swab
- A pair of nonsterile gloves
- Gauze covered cotton wool ball.

R Reposition patient accordingly

S State of patient.

ACE TIPS

- Ask the patient if they are in any pain before you touch them

- Ask the patient if they have any known **drug allergies**

Prior to procedure

- Explain to patient:
  - The benefits and side effects of the medication that you intend to administer
  - General implications of intramuscular injections, i.e., discomfort/pain, local infection and bruising, rarely nerve or blood vessel damage by needle
- Check patient's drug chart for:
  - Drug and dose to be injected
  - Correct prescription of drug, e.g., valid signature of prescribing doctor

- Time of day drug is to be administered (if specified)
- Any documented patient *allergies*
- Confirm drug and expiry date with another health professional
- Determine injection site:
  - *Ventrogluteal* (gluteus medius muscle) – most common site
  - *Dorsogluteal* (gluteus maximus muscle)
  - *Deltoid* (deltoid muscle)
  - *Vastus lateralis* (vastus lateralis muscle)

Procedure
- Wash hands and put on gloves.
- Check injection site for irregularities or infection.
- Draw up medication into syringe using green needle.
- Cleanse skin using an alcohol swab and allow to dry.
- Remove needle carefully from syringe and discard in sharps bin.
- Attach new blue or green needle to syringe.
- Warn patient of upcoming injection.
- Stretch the skin over the injection site and, with other hand, rapidly insert two thirds of the needle perpendicular to the skin.
- Slightly draw back upon the syringe to make certain that you have not penetrated a vein.
- Inject medication at a slow pace (e.g., 10 ml/s).
- Withdraw needle and syringe and dispose in sharps bin immediately.
- Apply gentle pressure over injection site with cotton wool ball.
- Check patient for signs of distress or anaphylaxis.
- Remove gloves and wash hands.

Finishing off
- Sign the drug chart and document procedure in patient notes.
- Advise patient to contact a member of staff if they feel unwell.
- Thank patient.
- Wash hands.

Subcutaneous Injection

Examiner's Instruction

"Mr Paul Shetland requires a heparin injection. Draw up the medication as prescribed and deliver the medication via the injection pad on the patients arm. Document the procedure."

ACE TIPS

- Ensure for a subcutaneous injection that the patients skin is pulled into a fold prior to giving the injection

- Be aware of the signs of anaphylaxis

Wh Wash hands

I Introduce yourself and identify patient (use their ID bracelet)

S Summarise procedure to patient and ask if they have any questions

P Permission – gain verbal consent

E Expose the injection site

E Equipment:
- Patient's drug chart
- Medication to be injected
- 10 ml syringe of appropriate size
- 25G (orange) needle and 21G (green) needle
- Alcohol swab
- A pair of nonsterile gloves

R Reposition patient accordingly

S State of patient.

ACE TIPS

- Ask the patient if they are in any pain before you touch them

- Ask the patient if they have any known **drug allergies**

Prior to procedure

- Explain to patient:
  - The benefits and side effects of the medication that you intend to administer
  - General complications of subcutaneous injections, i.e., discomfort, local infection and bruising

- Check patient's drug chart for:
  - Drug and dose to be injected
  - Correct prescription of drug, e.g., valid signature of prescribing doctor
  - Time of day drug is to be administered (if specified)
  - Any documented patient *allergies*
- Confirm drug and expiry date with another health professional
- Determine injection site:
  - Limbs – outer aspect of upper arms/anterior aspect of thighs
  - Abdomen – between the costal margins and iliac crests.

Procedure
- Wash hands and put on gloves
- Check injection site for irregularities or infection.
- Draw up medication into syringe using green needle.
- Remove needle carefully from syringe and discard in sharps bin.
- Attach orange needle to syringe.
- Cleanse skin using an alcohol swab and allow to dry.
- Warn patient of upcoming injection.
- Pinch an inch of skin gently to form a fold with one hand. With the other, rapidly insert the needle at 90 degrees into the fold of skin.
- Inject the medication at a slow pace (e.g. 10 ml/s).
- Withdraw needle and syringe and dispose in sharps bin immediately.
- Check patient for signs of distress or anaphylaxis.
- Remove gloves and wash hands.

Finishing off
- Sign the drug chart and document procedure in patient notes.
- Advise patient to contact a member of staff if they feel unwell.
- Thank patient.
- Wash hands.

Urine Dipstick

Examiner's Instruction

"You are working in a GP surgery and you have been asked to dip stick Miss Samantha Hat's urine and report your findings to the examiner."

* Wash hands using the 7-stage technique.
* Equipment:
  * A pair of nonsterile gloves
  * Urine sample pot
  * Urine reagent test strip and (dipstick) bottle?

Procedure

* Put on gloves.
* Check the date of the reagent strips.
* Unscrew the caps off both the urine and the dipstick bottle.
* Select a urine test strip from the dipstick box.
* Dip the urine test strip in the urine, ensuring that all the reagents are fully immersed.
* Submerge for 2–3 seconds and remove carefully, wiping any excess urine on the side of the specimen pot.
* Ensure you hold the reagent strip at right angles to the reagent strip container.

- Follow manufacturers instructions as to how long to wait for the reactions on the strip to occur. This is approximately 30–60 seconds.
- Hold the reagent strip against the colour chart on the reagent strip container and compare any colour changes on the reagent strip against those on the colour chart.
- State your findings to the examiner.
- Dispose of used reagent stick in clinical waste.
- Remove your gloves and wash your hands.
- Send sample for urine microscopy, culture and sensitivity if necessary.

Hand Washing

Examiner's instruction

"Demonstrate a 7-stage hand wash."

The 7-stage hand washing technique is relevant for washing with both soap and with alcohol – the same range of motions should be used in order to reach all areas of the hands. This technique should take approximately 30 seconds.

- Remove all watches and items of jewellery, and roll sleeves up to elbow. Watches and Jewellery should be put in your pocket or not worn, as you must not put these back on after hand washing otherwise you recontaminate your hands.

Procedure

Wet hands and apply soap or alcohol to hands.

Step 1: Rub hands together palm to palm.

Step 2: Place palm of one hand over the back of the other and interlock fingers and rub. Swap hands.

Step 3: Rub hands palm to palm with interlocking fingers.

Step 4: Rub the backs of the fingers of each hand into the palms of the opposite hand

Step 5: Grab thumb of one hand with the other hand and rub in a rotational manner. Swap hands.

Step 6: Rub fingers of each hand into the palms of the other hand. Swap hands.

Step 7: Rub each wrist with the opposite hand. Swap wrists.

After washing:

- Rinse hands thoroughly with finger tips in an upwards direction to ensure you do not recontaminate.

- Turn off the taps using elbows or feet.

- Dispense hand towel with your elbow (if too short to reach with elbow you will need to dispense the hand towel prior to washing your hands, ensure this does not touch any area of the sink).

- Dry hands thoroughly from finger tips down.

- Dispose of hand towel in clinical waste bin using the foot pedal to open the bin.

Nasogastric Tube Insertion

Examiner's instruction

*"You are working on a surgical ward and you have been asked to insert a **wide bore** nasogastric tube into Mr Jones prior to surgery. Please insert the nasogastric tube into the mannequin, as if they were a real patient."*

ACE TIPS

- Ensure you identify that you have the correct patient, even when being asked to insert an NG tube into a mannequin.

- Ensure you talk through the procedure as if you were doing it on a real patient.

- Ensure you follow hospital policy regarding the testing of the NG tube once it is inserted.

Placement of a nasogastric (NG) tube is a common procedure in both surgical and medical wards and is an essential skill for all foundation scheme doctors. Typically, insertion of an NG tube will be a procedural OSCE station in final year examinations. Insertion of an NG tube enables you to (1) drain gastric contents; (2) decompress the stomach; (3) obtain a specimen of gastric contents; or (4) introduce a passage into the GI tract (e.g., to allow nasogastric feeding).

In the vast majority of cases, NG tube placement occurs without incident; however, there is a risk that the tube can become misplaced in the mouth, upper oesophagus or lungs during insertion (or move out of the stomach at a later stage). Misplacement of an NG tube can have serious consequences for a patient. Therefore, it is of paramount importance that you are aware of methods to demonstrate the correct position of an NG tube. There are many guidelines of how to correctly insert a nasogastric tube – therefore you should familiarise yourself with the local guidelines of wherever you will be working as a junior doctor.

Typically in such OSCE stations you will be provided with a short clinical summary of the case, an appropriate mannequin and the necessary equipment to insert an NG tube.

Wh Wash hands

I Introduce yourself and identify the patient

S Summarise the procedure to the patient – including the indication for doing the procedure, what will happen and any potential complications. It is also good idea to arrange a method of signalling to enable the patient to request the procedure to proceed more slowly or stop. Ask if the patient has any questions

P Permission – gain the patients permission for doing the procedure

E Exposure of patient – expose the patients epigastric region

R Reposition the patient in a semirecumbent position

S State of patient. As with any procedure, it is always important to perform an appropriate clinical assessment of the patient.

Equipment

You should check that you have the appropriate equipment:

- Sterile 50 ml catheter tipped syringe
- Water soluble lubricant or sterile water (depending on local policy)
- Appropriate pH indicator strips (range 0–6 with half point gradations)
- Appropriate NG tube (i.e., wide bore tube)
- Indelible marker
- Tape
- Emesis basin
- Cup of water and straw
- Apron
- Eye protection (consider use)
- Sterile gloves, nonsterile gloves.

Procedure

Determination of the length of nasogastric tube required

- Determine the desired length of the NG that has to be inserted. There are many methods doing this. One such method is to place the tip of the tube against the patient's epigastrium, pass the tube behind the ear, over the top of the ear and to the tip of the patient's nostril.
- Mark this position with an indelible marker.

Insertion of nasogastric tube

- Depending on local policy, consider lubricating the patients nasal passage with water-soluble lubricant or sterile water.
- Pass the nasogastric tube into the nasal meatus and advance in a steady unhurried manner.
- If the patient can cooperate, request that when the tip of the tube is felt in the throat they should start to swallow; use the glass of water with a straw to aid this. Tilt the chin downward slightly at the same time.
- Continue to pass the tube until the required length has been inserted.
- Secure the NG tube with tape to the cheek.

ACE TIPS

- If obstruction is encountered, withdraw slightly then advance the NG tube at a slightly different angle. Gentle rotation of the tube can be helpful.

- Never force the NG tube. Withdraw the tube immediately if the patient demonstrates any signs of respiratory distress.

- Depending on the clinical condition, you may encourage the patient to swallow (e.g. sip water through a straw) and advance the NG tube as the patient swallows. Swallowing enhances the passage of the NG tube into the oesophagus.

Determination of placement of nasogastric tube

- This will depend on the local guidelines of the healthcare trust for whom you are working.
- One method for checking the placement of a nasogastric tube is by aspirating a sample with a 50 ml catheter-tipped syringe. Test the pH of the aspirate with appropriate pH paper. Gastric contents should have a pH ≤4. It is important that the resulting colour change is easily distinguishable.

ACE TIPS

- The most accurate method for confirming the correct placement of a NG tube is radiography. However X-rays are not required routinely to confirm correct placement. If it is not possible to obtain an aspirate or if the pH of the gastric contents is above 4 then an X-ray is required. Confirmation of correct position on a CXR should include: (1) a subdiaphragmatic location of the NG tube tip and (2) the NG tube should be clearly separate from the airway in its descent through the thorax into the abdomen. If you are unable to see the NG tube tip clearly below the diaphragm, do not allow the NG tube to be used until the X-ray has been reviewed by a senior doctor.

- The "whoosh" test, which involves the use of a syringe to push a small volume of air down the NG tube whilst listening for the sounds by a stethoscope, is usually not recommended.

- If there is **any** query about the position of the NG tube – no feeding or administration of any medication should take place.

- One of the limitations of testing pH is that stomach pH can be affected by medication (e.g., antacid medication), therefore you should always enquire if the patient is on any medication.

- Checking for the placement of a NG tube should always take place:

  - After initial insertion

  - Before administering each feed

  - Before giving medication via the NG tube

  - At least once daily during continuous feeds

  - Following any episode of vomiting or coughing

  - If you suspect the nasogastric tube has moved (e.g., loose tape or the tube appears longer).

Secure the nasogastric tube

- Anchor the tube securely to the patient's nose and cheek, keeping it out of their field of vision.

Finishing off

- Thank the patient.
- Correctly dispose of clinical waste.
- Wash your hands.

Document:

- Date and time of procedure
- Indication for insertion
- Type of tube used
- Distance tube inserted (if appropriate)
- The nature of the aspirate
- Methods used to check location of the tube insertion
- Any procedural comments.

Male Bladder Catheterisation

Examiner's instruction

"This model represents a man who requires catheterisation due to being in urinary retention. Catheterise the model and record the procedure."

ACE TIPS

- Ensure you maintain a sterile field throughout this procedure.

- Ensure you check that all medication, diluents etc. are correct and in date.

- Some hospital areas perform this procedure with a single glove technique; it is therefore important you are familiar different ways of performing this skill.

- Be aware of the patient's privacy at all times.

- Be aware of the patient's comfort at all times.

Wh Wash hands

I Introduce yourself and identify patient (use their ID bracelet)

S Summarise the purpose of catheterisation and explain the procedure; ask the patient if they have any questions

P Permission gain verbal consent

"Hello, my name is . . . and I am a medical student. Can I just check your name please? I would like to put a tube into your bladder by passing it through the opening of your penis. This will make it easier for you to empty your bladder and helps to inform me of how much urine you make. I will put in anaesthetic to minimise any discomfort. Is that OK? Do you have any questions?"

E Equipment:
- Apron
- A clean trolley
- A 14–16 g French Foley catheter
- A catheterisation pack : including s sterile drape, gallipot, and guaze.
- Saline solution (10 ml) check it is in date
- Lidocaine 2% gel in a pre-filled syringe, check it is in date
- A catheter bag
- Sterile examination gloves
- Sterile surgical gloves
- Distilled water (10 ml) and syringe.

R Reposition patient

S State of patient (well/unwell).

ACE TIPS

Ask the patient if they are in any pain before you touch them

Procedure

- Wash your hands using the 7-stage technique.
- Open the catheter pack onto the trolley and lay out the sterile field.
- Confirm the name and expiry date of the saline solution and pour the solution into the sterile pot.
- Open up the equipment into the sterile field: catheter bag, lidocaine gel and gloves into the sterile filed ensuring no contamination.
- Wash hands or use cleaning gel.
- Put on sterile gloves using the appropriate techniques ensuring not to touch the external side of the gloves.
- Put on sterile examination gloves.
- Open the drape provided in the catheter pack.
- Create a hole in the middle of the drape.
- Place the drape above the patients penis.
- Make a sling with the gauze and use this to hold the penis up with your nondominant hand.
- Soak the rest of the gauze or cotton wool in the saline solution and clean the meatus. Use single strokes away from the meatus. Make sure the foreskin is retracted.
- Warning the patient first that there maybe some discomfort Anesthetise the urethra by inserting the lidocaine gel.
- Tell the examiner you would wait up to 5 minutes for the anaesthetic to work.
- Remove the sterile examination gloves without contaminating the pair underneath.
- Connect the urine bag to the catheter.
- Carefully open the catheter tip, ensuring not to touch the catheter.
- Create another sling to hold the penis.
- Warn the patient that they may feel pressure but it should not be painful.
- Insert the catheter into the urethra.
- Once you have reached the bladder, urine should pass into the catheter bag. Continue to advance the catheter another couple of centimetres to ensure it is in the bladder.
- Inflate the balloon with appropriate volume of distilled water. Explain to the patient you are going to do this, and ask them to tell you if they feel any discomfort.
- Gently retract the catheter until you feel resistance.
- Reposition the foreskin.
- Remove the drape and cover the patient.
- Hang the catheter bag on an appropriate stand.

Finishing off

- Thank patient
- Cover them up
- Wash hands

Record the:
* Volume of urine in the catheter bag
* Dipstick the urine
* Problems faced during the procedure
* Type and size of the catheter, batch/reference number of catheter
* Volume of water injected into the balloon
* Date and time of the catheterisation
* That catheterisation was performed using an aseptic technique.

Female Catheterisation

Examiner's Instruction

"This model represents a lady who requires catheterisation due to being in urinary retention. Catheterise the model and record the procedure."

> ### ACE TIPS
>
> • Ensure you maintain a sterile field throughout this procedure.
>
> • Ensure you check that all medication, diluents etc. are correct and in date.
>
> • Some hospital areas perform this procedure with a single glove technique; it is therefore important you are familiar different ways of performing this skill.
>
> • Be aware of the patient's privacy at all times.
>
> • Be aware of the patient's comfort at all times.

Wh Wash hands

I Introduce yourself and identify patient (use their ID bracelet)

S Summarise the purpose of catheterisation and explain the procedure; ask the patient if they have any questions

P Permission – gain verbal consent

"Hello, my name is . . . and I am a . . . Year Medical Student. Can I check your name please? I have been asked to catheterize you today, which means putting this narrow tube into your bladder. This will make it much more comfortable for you to empty your bladder and help to inform me how much urine you are passing. Do you have any questions? I will use a local anaesthetic to minimise any discomfort. Is this OK?"

E Equipment:

- Apron
- *A clean trolley*
- A *female* urinary catheter
- A catheterisation pack: including sterile drape, gallipot, and gauze.
- Saline solution (10 ml); check it is in date
- Lidocaine 2% gel in a pre-filled syringe; check it is in date
- A catheter bag
- Sterile examination gloves
- Sterile surgical gloves
- Distilled water (10 ml) and syringe.

R Reposition patient

S State of patient (well/unwell).

> ### ACE TIPS
>
> Ask the patient if they are in any pain before you touch them

1

Prior to procedure

- Clean the trolley with alcohol and allow to dry.
- Put on an apron.
- Open the catheter pack carefully and prepare the sterile field.
- Open the sachet of cleaning solution and pour carefully into the sterile plastic bowl, without touching the bowl.
- Open the catheter, catheter bag, lidocaine gel and gloves into the sterile filed ensuring no contamination.
- Draw up sterile water into a 10 ml syringe and place *outside* sterile field of trolley.

Procedure

- Illuminate the genitals to aid your view.
- Wash hands or use cleaning gel.
- Don *both* pairs of sterile gloves correctly, i.e., without touching outside of glove.
- Open out the drape and make a hole in it.
- Place the drape over the female genitals.
- Soak the gauze and swab one side of the labia majora, wiping downwards. Dispose of the swab, soak another one and repeat on the opposite side, again wiping downwards.
- Repeat as above with fresh swabs to clean the labia minora.
- Warning the patient first that there maybe some discomfort, insert approximately 15 ml of anaesthetic gel using the pre-filled syringe.
- Wait up to 5 minutes for the anaesthetic to work.
- Remove outer pair of gloves without contaminating underneath pair and discard.
- Attach catheter to catheter bag (some hospitals attach the catheter bag after insertion of the catheter).
- Open the inner wrapping surrounding the catheter tip, making sure not to touch the tip.
- Insert the catheter into the urethral orifice, warning the patient first. Using an *aseptic non-touch technique*, gently advance the catheter into the urethra whilst removing the wrapping, thus not touching the catheter itself with your gloves.
- Insert as far as the bifurcation of the catheter.
- Slowly inject the appropriate amount of sterile water into the side tube to inflate the balloon. Explain to the patient you are going to do this and ask them to tell you if they feel any discomfort.
- Once full, gently retract the catheter until resistance is felt (the inflated balloon against the bladder neck).
- Remove the drape cover from the patient ensure their privacy is maintained by replacing the sheet over them.
- Ensure the catheter bag is correctly positioned to allow drainage of urine.
- Take off gloves, wash your hands.

Finishing off

- Thank the patient
- Cover them up
- Wash your hands
- Document in the patient's notes:
  - Residual volume of urine
  - Any complications encountered
  - Type and size of catheter used, and reference/batch number of the catheter
  - Amount of water used to inflate the balloon
  - Date and time of procedure
  - That the procedure was done under aseptic conditions
- If required, dipstick urine and/or send a sample for microscopy, culture and sensitivity.

● Suturing

Examiner's instruction

"You are working in Accident and Emergency. You have been asked to see Mr Philip Toms who has had an accident at work causing a laceration to his arm, which requires suturing. Speak to the examiner as if they are the patient and demonstrate your suturing skills on the skin pad."

> **ACE TIPS**
>
> Ensure you correctly identify the patient even if you asked to speak to the examiner and suture a model

Wh Wash your hands

I Introduce yourself and identify patient (use their ID bracelet)

S Summarise what you would like to do and ask patient if they have any questions

P Permission – gain verbal consent

"Hello, my name is ... and I am a medical student. Can I just check your name please? I would like to put stitches in your wound by passing a needle and thread through it to hold the skin together, helping it heal. I will put in anaesthetic to minimise any discomfort. Is that OK? Do you have any questions?"

E Equipment:
- A pair of nonsterile gloves
- A suture pack
  - Toothed forceps
  - Needle holder
  - Non-toothed forceps
- Cotton wool gauze
- Antiseptic solution
- A needle and syringe containing 1% lidocaine solution
- Scissors
- Dressing

R Reposition the wound so it is most accessible

S State of patient (well/unwell).

Prior to procedure
- Put on a pair of sterile gloves, making sure not to touch the outer parts of the gloves.
- Using the toothed forceps, separate the margins of the wound and inspect for any debris.
- Clean the wound using antiseptic solution soaked in gauze cotton wool.

Local anaesthetic
- Anaesthetise the wound with lidocaine 1% – administer the maximum dose of 3 mg/kg.
- This may be used with adrenaline to increase the duration of the effect. Adrenaline should not be used when suturing the hands, feet, ears, nose or penis.

- Warn the patient that they may feel a stinging sensation and that lignocaine may have adverse effects such as paraesthesia, anxiety or convulsions.
- Begin by puncturing the skin 1 cm from the wound, and drawing up on the syringe to make sure you have not punctured a vessel.
- Inject all around the wound.
- Wait up to 5 minutes for the anaesthetic to take effect.

Procedure

- Pick up the needle two thirds from the end using the needle holder. Use the non-toothed forceps to manoeuvre the position of the needle. Ensure the needle-end is pointing towards yourself.

> **ACE TIPS**
>
> Never hold the needle with your fingers

- Use the toothed forceps to grip the edges of the wound. This will make it easier to feed the needle into the skin.
- Hold the edge of the wound with toothed forceps.
- Feed the needle into the skin towards you and then pull it up through the middle of the wound. Use the non-toothed forceps to pull the rest of the needle and suture through.
- Transfer the needle from the forceps to the needle holder. Feed the needle through the opposite edge of the wound and puncture the skin 0.5 cm away from the wound edge.
- Again, use the toothed forceps to pull the needle and suture through.
- Wrap the long piece of thread around the needle holder twice. Then use the needle holder to grab hold of the short tail. Pull the tail through towards you and push the longer piece away from you.
- Repeat this process in the opposite direction. Wrap the longer piece around the needle holder once, grab hold of the short tail and pull the piece through away from you and the longer piece towards you.
- Repeat this process once more, pulling the short tail towards you.
- Cut both ends of the knot.
- Suture across the line of the wound, with each suture separated approx 0.5–1 cm apart.
- Dispose of the needle into the sharps box.

Finishing off

- Clean the wound and apply a dressing.
- Tell the patient when to come to get sutures removed – roughly:
  - Foot: 10–14 days
  - Leg: 1 week
  - Trunk: 1 week
  - Scalp: 5 days
  - Face: 3–4 days
- Thank patient
- Make sure patient is comfortable and offer to help cover them up
- Remove gloves and dispose of in clinical waste
- Wash hands.

Scrubbing Up for Theatre

At the beginning of the station, tell the examiner you would wear:
- Surgical scrubs
- Clogs
- A theatre hat with all your hair neatly tucked underneath
- A mask securely fastened over the nose and mouth
- Short nails with all jewellery removed.

Equipment
- Surgical gown
- Surgical gloves
- Cleansing solution – chlorohexidine gluconate or providone iodine.

Procedure
- Open the surgical pack onto a clean surface using an aseptic technique, i.e., do not touch the inside of the pack with your hands.
- Open a sterile gloves packet into your sterile field without touching it.
- Turn the water taps on to a comfortable temperature.
- Rinse both your arms from hand to elbow
- Lather the nailbrush in cleansing solution. Use the brush to wash your nails until they are clean.
- Use the sponge to scrub your hands using the 7-stage technique. Continue up the back and front of the forearm, right up to the elbow.
- Rinse from finger tips to elbow.
- Make sure you do not touch the taps. Use the back of your elbows to close them.
- If this is your first scrub of the day, it should be 5 minutes long.
- Subsequent scrubs should be 3 minutes long.
- Dry your hands and arms using the sterile towel.
- Using a sterile aseptic technique put on the gown touching only the inside.
- When you put your arms into the sleeve, be sure not to put your hand through the cuff.
- Ask somebody who is not surgically scrubbed up to tie your gown up for you at the back.
- Put your gloves on, making sure to touch only the inside of the glove.
- You are now ready for theatre. Be careful not to touch anything that is not in your sterile held. Keep your hands together in front of you.

◉ Blood Pressure Measurement

Wh Wash hands

I Introduce yourself and identify patient

S Summarise that you would like to take their blood pressure

P Permission

"Hello, my name is . . . and I am a medical student. Can I just check your name please? I would like to take your blood pressure by inflating a cuff round your arm and listening to your pulse as I deflate the cuff. It may feel a bit tight but it should not be painful. Is that OK?"

E Expose the arm by either rolling up the sleeve or taking shirt off

E Equipment – blood pressure sphygmomanometer and cuff; stethoscope

R Reposition the patient lying supine or sitting up

S State of patient.

ACE TIPS

Ask the patient if they are in pain before you touch them

Estimate the blood pressure

- Tie the cuff approximately 2 cm above the antecubital fossa with arrow of the cuff placed above the artery.
  - The brachial artery is about one third of the way across the antecubital fossa from the median side.
- The cuff must be at approximately the level of the heart.
- To estimate the systolic blood pressure, inflate the cuff until you can no longer feel the radial pulse.
- Deflate cuff and wait 20 seconds.

Accurately measure the blood pressure

- Place diaphragm of the stethoscope over brachial artery pulse.
- Reinflate cuff to a pressure of 20–30 mmHg higher than the blood pressure from palpation.
- Deflate cuff at a rate of 2–3 mmHg/s.
- Listen to when you first hear consistent heart sounds.
  - This is Korotokov sound I and indicates the systolic blood pressure.
- As you continue to deflate the cuff, the sound may muffle then disappear.
- This is called Korotokov IV and V and indicates diastolic pressure.

Assess for postural hypotension

- Tell the patient to stand up.
- Wait 2 minutes more and take the standing blood pressure.

You are looking for a fall in systolic pressure of greater than 20 mmHg between lying and standing to indicate postural hypotension.

Finishing off

- Thank patient
- Wash hands
- Cover the patient up
- Present and summarise to the examiner.

Performing a 12-Lead Electrocardiogram

Examiner's instruction

"You working on a critical care ward and have been asked to perform a 12-lead ECG on Mr. Ted Brent, a 25 year old patient. Present your findings to the examiner."

ACE TIPS

- Ensure you are familiar with the ECG machine you will be examined on
- Ensure you know common ECG rhythms

Wh Wash hands

I Introduce yourself and identify patient (use their ID bracelet)

S Summarise the purpose of an electrocardiogram (ECG) and explain the procedure (ask if any questions)

P Permission – gain verbal consent

E Expose the chest and ankles of the patient

E Equipment:
- ECG machine
- 6 chest leads (V1–V6)
- 4 limb leads (red, yellow, green, black)
- 10 adhesive pads

R Reposition the patient sitting at 45 degrees

S State of patient (well/unwell).

Procedure

Place 10 adhesive pads in the correct positions in order to attach the chest and limb leads:

- Chest leads:
    V1 – fourth intercostal space, right sternal edge
    V2 – fourth intercostal space, left sternal edge
    V3 – midway between V2 and V4
    V4 – fifth intercostal space, left midclavicular line (apex area)
    V5 – left anterior axillary line, in the same horizontal level as V4
    V6 – left midaxillary line, in the same horizontal level as V4.

- Limb leads

  Red – right shoulder/upper arm

  Yellow – left shoulder/upper arm

  Green – left ankle/pelvis

  Black – right ankle/pelvis.

- If performing an ECG on a male patient, it may be necessary to shave their chest hair if it is found to interfere with the ECG trace.
- Once the pads are attached, attach each of the appropriate leads.
- Ask the patient to lie as still as possible.
- Turn on the ECG machine and check that it is correctly calibrated (press 1 mV – the height of the mark formed should be ten small squares).
- When you can visualise a clear reading on the monitor, begin recording an ECG trace.
- If this attempt does not generate an adequate trace, retry until a clear printout is produced.
- Tear off the ECG printout.
- Remove the leads and pads from the patient and help them dress.

Finishing off

- Label the printout with:
  - Patient's name
  - Patient's date of birth
  - Hospital number
  - Date and time of the procedure
  - Whether or not the patient was experiencing chest pain at the time of recording.
- Ensure the ECG is reviewed by a qualified doctor.
- Ask if the patient has any questions.
- Thank patient.
- Cover them up.
- Wash hands.

Interpreting an Electrocardiogram

Examiner's instruction

"Please present this ECG."

Common OSCE cases

Essential to recognize:

- Myocardial infarction
- Atrial fibrillation
- Ventricular tachycardia
- Ventricular fibrillation

Should be able to recognize:

- Pulmonary embolism
- Hyperkalemia
- Digoxin toxicity
- Sinus tachycardia
- First degree heart block
- Second degree heart block
- Bivesicular block
- Complete heart block
- Left ventricular hypertrophy
- Left bundle branch block

Prior to procedure

Take patient details:

- Name
- Age
- Date of assessment.

The rhythm strip

The rhythm strip is recorded at the bottom of the trace, usually from L2. Before attempting to interpret the individual lead traces, much information can be gathered from the rhythm strip.

Determine the heart rate

- Count the number of large squares within an RR interval.
- Heart rate (HR) = 300/ no. of large squares.
- Record both the upper and lower limits of the HR if there is variation.

> **ACE TIPS**
>
> - Each small square is 1 mm wide, and represents 40 milliseconds. 5 small squares equal 1 large square.
>
> - On a 12-lead ECG, there is a quick, simple way to determine the rate:
>
>   No. of QRS complexes × 6
>
> - This is very useful when the rhythm is irregular.

The intervals

- Now count the number of small squares from the beginning of the P wave to the R wave (PR interval). This is usually 3–5 small squares (0.12–0.20 s). Prolonged PR interval is greater than 1 large square.
- Determine the QRS interval (usually 2–3 small squares: 0.08–0.12 s).
- Record both the upper and lower limits of the intervals if there is variation.

The rhythm

Sinus rhythm

- Depolarisation begins in the sinoatrial node (SAN), and is evident when a P wave is followed by a QRS complex, and the PR interval is normal.
- An isolated decrease in the RR interval in an otherwise regular sinus rhythm strip is called an "ectopic beat". If the ectopic QRS complex is wide, this is known as a ventricular ectopic. These can turn into ventricular fibrillation.
- Sinus tachycardia = sinus rhythm + heart rate greater than 100 bpm
- Sinus bradycardia = sinus rhythm + heart rate less than 60 bpm

Supraventricular tachycardia

- Depolarisation begins within the atrium, away from the sinoatrial node, and the heart rate is greater than 100 bpm.
- Atrial tachycardia – the p wave appears abnormal.
- Atrial flutter:
  - Several P waves are seen preceding every QRS complex.
  - The P waves are characteristically "saw toothed".
  - Two saw toothed P waves preceding each QRS complex is known as atrial flutter with 2 : 1 block.
- Junctional tachycardia:
  - The P waves may be absent – hidden within the QRS complexes.
  - The rhythm is regular (note: different from atrial fibrillation).
- Wolff–Parkinson–White syndrome:
  - Extra electrical connection between the atrium and the ventricle
  - The PR interval is narrowed.
  - The QRS complex appears widened and demonstrates a slurred upstroke (delta wave).

Atrial fibrillation

- Disorganized electrical activity occurs within the atrium.
- The P waves appear to be absent.
- The isoelectric line appears irregular.
- The RR interval is characteristically irregular.

Ventricular tachycardia (VT)

- Depolarisation begins within the ventricle, and the heart rate is greater than 100 bpm.
- The QRS complexes are **wide**.
- The RR intervals are regular.
- The chest leads are all positive or negative – known as concordance.

Ventricular fibrillation

- Disorganized electrical activity occurs within the ventricle.
- The QRS complexes are wide.
- The RR intervals are irregular.
- Fine ventricular fibrillation describes the ECG appearance when the QRS complexes seem unclear.

Heart block

There is a conduction defect within the AV node.

- First degree heart block – here the PR interval is consistently prolonged (greater than 1 large square).
- Second degree heart block:
  - Mobitz type 1 (Wenckebach phenomenon) – the PR interval appears to increase with each beat with an eventual dropped beat (a dropped beat is when a P wave is not followed by a QRS complex). This is usually benign.
  - Mobitz type 2 – the PR interval is consistently prolonged with a random dropped beat. This can develop into complete heart block
  - 2 : 1 block – 2 P waves precede 1 QRS complex
    3 : 1 block – 3 P waves preceded 1 QRS complex
    These can develop into complete heart block.

Causes of first and second degree heart block

- Normal variant
- Ischaemic heart disease
- Drugs – beta-blockers, digoxin

- Third degree heart block – complete heart block:
  - The atria and ventricles are depolarising independently.
  - The RR intervals are regular

- The distance between two P waves are regular,
- There is usually more than one P wave before each QRS complex.
- However, the PR interval is irregular.

Causes of complete heart block

- Fibrosis
- Ischaemic heart disease

The individual leads

The cardiac axis

- As the ventricles depolarise, electrical impulses run down the ventricles at various angles. The cardiac axis is the "average" angle at which the impulses travel.
- Assess the axis by inspecting the QRS complexes in Leads I (LI), II (LII) and III (LIII).
- There are only three interpretations to make – normal axis, left axis deviation and right axis deviation.
- Note: the isoelectric line will go up in a lead when the electrical signal is travelling towards the lead. So, for example, if the line goes up in lead I it means the electrical impulse is travelling towards lead I.
- If the line is half up and half down it means the electrical signal is travelling at 90 degrees to the lead.

ACE TIP

Quick guide to working out the axis:

- If both LI and LII point up, the axis is "normal"
- If LI points up and LII points down, this is left axis deviation
- If LI points down and LII points up, this is right axis deviation

Causes of left axis deviation

- Left anterior hemiblock
- Left ventricular hypertrophy
- Inferior myocardial infarction

Causes of right axis deviation

- Right ventricular hypertrophy
- Pulmonary embolism
- Anterolateral myocardial infraction

Ventricular hypertrophy (VH)

Left ventricular hypertrophy

* Inspect the R wave in chest lead 6 (V6) and the S wave in Chest lead 1 (V1)
    * The R wave in V6 is greater than 5 large blocks (25 mm)
    OR
    * The (S wave of V1) + (R wave in V6) is greater than 7 large blocks (35 mm)
* If left VH is suspected, look for evidence of strain to the left side of the heart, indicated by T wave inversion in V5 and V6.

Right ventricular hypertrophy

* In a normal ECG, there is a prominent S wave in V1. The presence of a prominent R wave in V1 suggests Right VH.
* If right VH is suspected, look for evidence of strain to the right side of the heart, indicated by T wave inversion in V2 and V3. Note that the T wave is normally inverted in V1.

Bundle Branch Block (BBB)

Electrical impulses enter the left and right bundle branches from the His bundles beneath the AV node. Consequent to a blocked bundle branch, electrical activity must travel down the ventricle muscle itself, resulting in a widening of the QRS complex. Only look for BBB if you found the QRS interval in the rhythm strip to be greater than the QRS upper limit (3 small squares).

* Assess for BBB by inspecting the QRS complexes in (V1) and (V6).
    * Do you see an "M" shape in VI – right BBB
    * Do you see an "M" shape in V6 – left BBB
    * Be careful in your assessment as it may not look like an obvious "M".

ACE TIP

New onset left bundle branch block may be a sign of infarction.

Note: you can not interpret the ST segment on T wave if you see an "M" in V6.

Causes of left bundle branch block

* Myocardial infarction
* Aortic stenosis
* Hypertension

Causes of right bundle branch block

* Normal variant
* Congenital heart disease
* Pulmonary embolism
* Cor pulmonale

Note: It can be difficult to distinguish between supraventricular tachycardia with bundle branch block and ventricular tachycardia as both have broad QRS complexes and fast heart rates.

Lead trace morphology

Take time to look now at the morphology of each P wave, Q wave, ST segment, and T wave in the limb and chest leads. With experience this will take only a few seconds.

The chest and limb leads are organized to look at different sides of the heart. Commit the list in the box to memory.

ACE TIPS

Do not assess the traces from each lead in a numerical order – instead, inspect the traces of the leads from the same side of the heart.

I, AvL, V5/6: these view the lateral side

II, III, AvF: these view the inferior side

V2, V3, V4: these view the anterior side

Anomalies to look for are listed below.

P waves

- P-mitrale: bifid P waves – suggests left atrial hypertrophy
- P-pulmonale: tall P waves – suggests right atrial hypertrophy.

QRS complex

- Pathological Q waves – seen following a myocardial infarction
- There is a negative deflection greater than 1 mm across and 2 mm deep.

ST segments

- Depressed below the isoelectric line – indicates ischaemia
- Elevated above the isoelectric line – indicates infarction
- Downsloping – digoxin toxicity (reverse tick sign).

ACE TIP

Watch out for the scenario of the young patient with chest pain and ST elevation. The ST elevation will often be saddle shaped and in multiple leads indicating pericarditis rather than infarction.

T waves

- Inverted – indicates ischemia (normally inverted V1 and AvR)
- Tall – indicates hyperkalaemia
- Flattened – indicates hypokalaemia.

Case presentations

Case 1

"Mr X is a 72-year-old gentleman who described episodes of dizziness and complained that his heart seemed to be racing. His GP decided to perform an ECG and then calls you for advice. His description is given below."

- Rhythm strip: his heart rate is approximately 120. The rhythm strip shows absent P waves, an irregular baseline and an irregular rhythm. The QRS complexes are not wide.
- Cardiac axis: the cardiac axis is not deviated.
- Ventricular hypertrophy: there is no evidence of ventricular hypertrophy.
- Lead trace morphology: there are no abnormalities in any of the P waves, or ST segments, and there is no evidence of any pathological Q waves. The T waves appear normal.

Summary

"This ECG demonstrates atrial fibrillation."

Case 2

"Mr Y is a 58-year-old gentleman who has type II diabetes and hypertension. He is brought into the A&E department with central chest pain, which is associated with nausea and SOB. An ECG was performed on arrival."

- Rhythm strip: His heart rate is approximately 100. The PR and QRS intervals are within the normal range. The trace shows sinus rhythm.
- Cardiac axis: the cardiac axis is deviated to the right
- Ventricular hypertrophy: there is no evidence of ventricular hypertrophy.
- Lead trace morphology: there are no abnormalities in any of the P waves. There is ST segment elevation in leads LII, LIII, and AvF, as well as ST depression in LI, AvL, V5 and V6. There is evidence of pathological Q waves, which may be old or new in LII and LIII. The T waves appear normal.

Summary

"This ECG demonstrates an inferior myocardial infarction with reciprocal changes in the lateral leads."

(Note: Beware the diabetic patient who presents feeling suddenly SOB but with no associated chest pain. It is not uncommon for diabetics to present with silent myocardial infarctions.)

Case 3

"Mrs A, age 81 presented following an episode of sharp chest pain located over the left side of her chest. The pain was associated with SOB. She has a past medical history of breast cancer, which she receives hormone therapy for. An ECG was performed and is described as follows:

- Rhythm strip: her heart rate is approximately 120. The PR interval is normal. The QRS interval is 0.16 second, and this is prolonged. The trace shows sinus rhythm.
- Cardiac axis: the cardiac axis is deviated to the right

- Ventricular hypertrophy: there is an R wave seen in V1 suggestive of right ventricular hypertrophy, as well as inverted t waves in V2 and V3, indicative of right ventricular strain.
- Bundle branch block: there is an M pattern in V1 consistent with right bundle branch block.
- Lead trace morphology: there are no abnormalities in any of the P waves, or ST segments. There appears to be a pathological Q wave in lead III.

Summary

"This ECG demonstrates sinus tachycardia, right axis deviation, right ventricular hypertrophy, right bundle branch block. There is also a pathological Q wave in lead III. These features are classic of a pulmonary embolism.

(Note: Most common ECG changes in pulmonary embolism are with sinus tachycardia alone.)

Case 4

"Mr G is a 67-year-old gentleman who has cardiac failure. He was admitted with peripheral oedema and SOB. He was started on spironolactone and lisinopril. A routine ECG was performed on the ward and is described below."

- Rhythm strip: his heart rate is approximately 75. The PR interval is normal. The QRS interval is 0.16 second, and this is prolonged. The trace shows sinus rhythm.
- Cardiac axis: the cardiac axis is not deviated.
- Ventricular hypertrophy: there is no evidence of ventricular hypertrophy.
- Bundle branch block: there is no evidence of BBB.
- Lead trace morphology: there are no abnormalities in any of the P waves, or ST segments, and there is no evidence of any pathological Q waves. The T waves appear peaked in several of the lead traces.

Summary

"This ECG demonstrates the changes associated with hyperkalaemia."

Case 5

"You are called to see Mrs H on the ward, a 74-year-old lady with known heart failure, who has been complaining of nausea and vomiting for the last 2 days, which is not controlled by antiemetics. She was admitted a week ago and was found to be in fast atrial fibrillation."

- Rhythm strip: her heart rate is approximately 30. The rhythm strip shows absent P waves, and an irregular rhythm. The QRS complexes are wide.
- Cardiac axis: the cardiac axis is not deviated.
- Ventricular hypertrophy: there is no evidence of ventricular hypertrophy.
- Bundle branch block: there is no evidence of BBB.
- Lead trace morphology: there are no abnormalities in any of the P waves, and there is no evidence of any pathological Q waves. The ST segments are down slopping, known as the reverse tick sign. The T waves appear normal.

Summary

"The ECG demonstrates AF with digoxin toxicity."

⚙ Explain How to Use a Peak Expiratory Flow Rate Meter

Examiner's instruction

"You are working in a GP surgery. The GP has asked you to explain and demonstrate how to use a peak flow meter to Hannah Pauls who has recently been diagnosed with asthma."

ACE TIPS

• Ensure you communicate clearly and concisely to the patient

• Demonstrate/explain the procedure then ask the patient to go through it with you to ensure they have understood the technique

---

Wh Wash hands

I Introduce yourself and identify patient

S Summarise what you would like to do and ask if patient has any questions

P Permission

"Hello, my name is ... and I am a medical student. Can I just check your name please? I would like to assess your lung function by asking you to blow into a mouthpiece for me. Is that OK? Do you have any questions?"

R Reposition patient

S State of patient (well/unwell).

• Ask the patient to explain what they already know about the condition they are being assessed for by using the peak expiratory flow rate (PEFR) meter – usually asthma or COPD

• Ask them if they have ever used a PEFR meter before, when they use it during the day, and ask them to demonstrate their technique to identify any errors in use.

Procedure

• Hand the patient the PEFR meter with a new mouthpiece attached and with the dial pointing to zero. Medical student may need to demonstrate first.

• The patient should ideally stand up

• "I would like you to take a deep breath in, put the mouthpiece into your mouth forming a tight seal and then to blow out as hard and as fast as possible, like you were blowing out some candles."

• Record the reading – repeat this 3 times and take the best value.

• Compare their best reading to their previous readings as written in their notes, and also compare to the chart of expected PEFR.

• Dispose of the mouth piece in the clinical waste bin.

Finishing off

- Thank patient
- Summarise what you have discussed
- Offer to answer any questions
- Consider arranging a follow up appointment to assess progress
- Provide yourself with a safety net by offering your medical expertise to the patient in case of any problems or concerns
- Offer the patient a leaflet regarding your topics of discussion.

⊙ Inhaler Technique

Examiner's instructions

"You are working in a GP surgery. The GP has asked you to see Anne Peters a recently diagnosed asthmatic to explain and demonstrate inhaler technique."

> **ACE TIPS**
>
> • Ensure you communicate clearly and concisely to the patient.
>
> • Demonstrate/explain the procedure then ask the patient to go through it with you to ensure they have understood the technique.

Wh Wash hands

I Introduce yourself and identify patient

S Summarise what you would like to do, ask if patient has any questions.

P Permission

  "A bronchodilator gives sudden relief during an asthma attack by opening up the airways and relaxing the muscles. Steroids help breathlessness over a longer period of time. I would like to demonstrate to you how to use an inhaler correctly. Is that OK?"

1 **E** Equipment – inhaler

R Reposition patient

S State of patient (well/unwell).

• Ask the patient what they know about their condition that requires an inhaler (usually asthma or COPD)

• Ask them what they understand about the medication they are being given through the inhaler.

Procedure

• Check the medication, even it is if a placebo it has a date on it.

• Begin by shaking the inhaler vigorously.

• Remove the cap from the mouthpiece.

• The patient should be sat in a upright position to aid distribution of the medication.

  "Keeping the inhaler upright in front of you, breath out, and as you breathe in, place the inhaler in your mouth, push down on the canister and continue to breathe in."

• You should only deliver one dose of medication at a time.

  "Remove the inhaler from your mouth, and hold your breath for 10 seconds. Then breathe out and wait about 1 minute before using the inhaler again."

• Watch the patient perform the technique.

- Those who have difficulty using a metered dose inhaler may wish to use a spacer device.
  - The inhaler is attached to the spacer. The canister is pushed down once for one dose.
  - From the opposite end of the spacer, the patient draws in a deep breath and holds their breath for about 10 seconds, then breathes out through the mouthpiece.
  - The patient can continue to breathe in and out through the spacer device without pressing the canister. Wait about 1 minute before releasing another dose in to the spacer.

Finishing off

- Thank patient
- Summarise what you have discussed
- Offer to answer any questions
- Consider arranging a follow up appointment to assess progress
- Provide yourself with a safety net by offering your medical expertise to the patient in case of any problems or concerns
- Offer the patient a leaflet regarding your topics of discussion.

⊙ Using a Nebuliser

Examiner's instruction

"You are working on a medical ward and you have been asked to administer a nebuliser to Mr Dan Potter who has exacerbation of his asthma."

ACE TIPS

- If you are giving the nebuliser via a mask ensure that you fit it properly to the patient.
- Ensure you read the drug chart thoroughly, and document when you have given the medication.
- You may also be asked to prescribe the nebuliser so ensure you able to do this.
- Ensure the air flow is set to the correct amount to deliver the medication.

Wh Wash your hands using the 7-stage technique

I Introduce yourself and identify patient (use their ID bracelet)

S Summarise what is involved and the intended purpose of a nebuliser, and ask the patient if they have any questions

P Permission – gain verbal consent

E Equipment:
- Nebuliser
- Mask or mouthpiece to administer drug
- Nebule containing medication required, e.g., salbutamol
- Diluent, e.g., sterile 0.9% saline
- Oxygen tubing.

R Reposition patient sitting upright

S State of patient.

ACE TIPS

Ask the patient if they have any known drug allergies

Prior to procedure
Explain to patient:

- The intended benefits and side effects of the medication that you intend to administer
- That a nebuliser is a method of administering a drug as an aerosol that the patient is required to breathe in via a mouthpiece/mask

- Warn the patient that the machine is noisy, there may be steam emitted from the mouthpiece/mask and that they will need to keep the mouthpiece/mask on for approximately 5–10 minutes.

Procedure

- Check patient's drug chart for:
  - Correct prescription of drug, e.g., valid signature of prescribing doctor
  - Drug and dose of drug to be administered
  - Any documented patient *allergies*.
- Sit the patient upright.
- Select the correct nebule containing the required medication and dose. In some hospitals two drugs can be administered simultaneously, e.g. salbutamol and ipatropium bromide.
- Check the drug and expiry date with another health professional.
- Fill the chamber of the nebuliser with the contents of the prescribed nebule.
- The total volume of the chamber should be approximately 5 ml so, if required, add an appropriate amount of diluent (normal saline only, *not* sterile water).
- Attach the chamber to the mask and air flow.
- Place the mask (or mouthpiece) over the patient's mouth; perhaps put the mask on after drawing up medication as chamber has to be attached to mask and air flow.
- Set the gas flow rate at 6–8 litres/minute – air should be used as the gas of choice to drive the nebuliser unless oxygen is specifically stated on the prescription (for instance in acute asthma).
- Ask the patient to relax and breathe through their mouth for the duration of administration, normally 5–10 minutes.

Finishing off

- After the nebuliser has administered the entire drug from the chamber, remove device from the patient and rinse the mask and chamber in warm soapy water. Dry with a disposable tissue.
- Sign drug chart and document procedure in patient's notes.
- Thank patient.
- Wash your hands.

Basic Life Support: Community Based

Examiners instruction

"A lady has collapsed in the street. Nobody else is around to assist you. Assess the situation and start the appropriate resuscitation."

ACE TIPS

- Ensure you are up to date with the current resuscitation council guidelines.

- Make sure, if safe to do so, you open the airway with a head tilt/chin lift manoeuvre not in any other way.

- Ensure the airway is open when delivering mouth to mouth.

- Know the rate per minute for chest compressions and perform them at this rate.

- Know what information to give when calling 999.

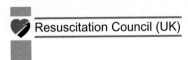 Resuscitation Council (UK)

Adult Basic Life Support

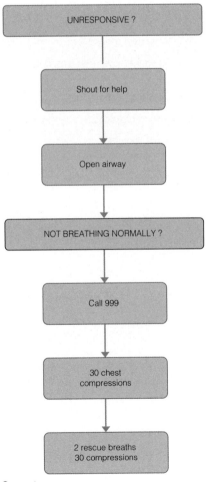

Adult Basic Life Support

Procedure

- Assess for any surrounding danger to yourself and the patient, such as fire, chemical spills, traffic, live electrical wires.
- Approach the patient.
- Assess level of responsiveness of the patient by gently shaking their shoulders and shouting in both ears.
- If no response from the patient, shout for help and follow the ABC approach.

The ABC approach

A – Airway

- Check for any obvious visible signs of obstruction such as vomit or debris.
- Remove loose fitting (but not well fitting) dentures.
- Perform *head tilt* and *chin lift* manoeuvre.
- If you suspect a C-spine injury, perform a *jaw thrust* manoeuvre instead.

B – Breathing

C – Circulation

- Assess these simultaneously – place your ear close to the patient's mouth whilst watching the patient's chest. Place your first 2 fingers to check for a pulse over the carotid pulse, remain here for 10 seconds.

  Look for movement of the chest wall indicating breathing.

  Listen for breath sounds.

  Feel for breath on your cheek and also a pulse under your fingers.

- If there are no signs of normal breathing or a circulation, get help – if there is nobody else around you may have to leave your patient to call 999.
- Immediately perform 30 chest compressions – place one hand over the centre of the patient's chest, place the other hand on top and interlock fingers. Arms should be straight and you should be vertically over the patient's chest, compressing the chest to a third of its depth. Compressions should be at a rate of 100 per minute
- Perform 2 ventilation breaths. Mouth to mouth ventilation maybe used when in the community.
- Continue a cycle of 30 compressions to every 2 effective breaths until the patient begins to breathe normally, help arrives or you become exhausted.

Extra component to basic life support station

- You may be presented with an automated external defibrillator (AED), which is now found in public areas. You may be asked to explain/ demonstrate its usage.
- An AED is a portable defibrillator that can assess for both ventricular fibrillation and ventricular tachycardia and provide a shock.

Paediatric Basic Life Support

Some important considerations

- An infant is a child under 1 year.
- A child is between 1 year and puberty.
- Lay rescuers should use a ratio of 30 compressions to 2 ventilations.

Procedure

- Assess for any surrounding danger to yourself and the patient, such as fire, chemical spills, traffic, live electrical wires.
- Approach the patient with care.
- Check the child's level of responsiveness by gently stimulating them and ask "are you all right?" Do not shake if you suspect cervical spine injury and immobilise the neck and spine.
- If the child responds by answering or moving then leave the child in the position you found them, checking their condition with regular review and summon help.
- If no response from the patient, shout for help and follow the ABC approach.

The ABC approach

A – Airway

- Open the airway using the *head tilt/chin lift* manoeuvre (if you suspect a C-spine injury, perform a *jaw thrust* manoeuvre instead). The blind finger sweep should not be used in children.
- In an infant the desirable degree of tilt is less than a child – the neutral position.
- If there is still difficulty opening the airway then try the jaw thrust technique.
- Assess patency of the airway:

  Look for chest and/or abdominal movement.

  Listen for breath sounds.

  Feel for breath.

- Look, listen and feel for no more than 10 seconds before deciding breathing is present or absent.

B – Breathing

- If the child *is breathing* then place them in the recovery position and check for continued breathing, ensuring help is on it's way.
- If the child *is not breathing* then give *five initial rescue breaths*. Seal your mouth around the mouth of a child, whilst pinching the nose, or around the mouth and nose for an infant.
- Blow steadily over 1–1.5 seconds looking for rising of the chest wall, taking a breath between rescue breaths to maximise oxygen deliverance.
- If there are difficulties achieving an effective breath then readjust your head tilt/chin lift position, and if this fails then adopt the jaw thrust method.
- Whilst performing rescue breaths note any cough or gag responses.

C – Circulation

- Check for signs of circulation, e.g., movement, coughing, normal breathing.
- *Check the pulse* (for no more than 10 seconds). In children feel the carotid artery but in infants feel the brachial or femoral artery.
- If you *can detect signs of circulation* then continue rescue breathing; place the child in the recovery position and reassess the child frequently.
- If you *cannot detect signs of circulation* or *absent pulse* or *slow pulse* (less than 60 per minute with poor perfusion) then start chest compressions.
- Combine and continue chest compressions with rescue breathing at a ratio of 15:2.
- Continue resuscitation until further help arrives, the child shows signs of life or you become exhausted.

Considerations

If only one rescuer is present, perform basic life support (BLS) for 1 minute then activate the EMS (emergency medical services) yourself. For an infant, you may be able to carry him or her whilst summoning help.

Activation of the EMS prior to commencing BLS by a lone rescuer is indicated if there is a witnessed sudden collapse. In this case, cardiac arrest is likely to be due to an arrhythmia and defibrillation is necessary.

Chest compressions

Position

The finger/thumb or hand position for all ages is one finger's breadth above the xiphisternum.

- **Infants**: use the hand-encircling method (two or more rescuers). The lone rescuer should compress the sternum with the tips of two fingers. Compress to one third of the depth of the infant's chest.
- **Children**: place the heel of one hand over the lower third of the sternum, depressing the sternum by approximately one third of the depth of the chest.

Rate

The compression rate for all ages is 100 per minute.

Examiners instructions

"An unconscious patient has been brought into the Accident and Emergency Department. Assess the situation and commence appropriate resuscitation."

Common OSCE cases

- You will need to be able to recognise the different advanced life support (ALS) algorithms.
- The most commonly used defibrillator used in hospitals is the biphasic defibrillator.

British resuscitation algorithm

The ALS algorithm begins by following the BLS algorithm – i.e., assessing for danger, following the ABC approach and performing CPR.

- Continue CPR until a defibrillator and help arrives.
- Once the defibrillator has arrived, open the pad packs and apply the pads to the patient's chest.
- Continue CPR throughout.
- One should be stuck at the right of the sternum, the other over the area of the apex.
- Connect the defibrillator and switch on the machine.
- Select "LEAD II" to assess the rhythm of the patient.
- Check if a pulse is palpable.

Shockable rhythms

- Pulseless ventricular tachycardia:
  - Rapid, regular, broad complex rhythm
  - Usually monomorphic
  - If polymorphic, known as *torsades de pointes.*
- Ventricular fibrillation (VF):
  - Irregular waveform with random rate, frequency and amplitude
  - No QRS complexes identifiable.

Follow the left hand loop of the algorithm.

- Charge the defibrillator to the required energy level as stated in the defibrillator manual.
- Warn the team to *"stand clear"* and look to ensure that there are no members of the team in contact with the patient, the bed or the trolley. Actively check the top, middle and bottom of the patient. Call *"oxygen away"* to inform the person ventilating the patient to remove any oxygen source. Warn the team that that machine is ready to shock and *deliver shock.*
- *Immediately resume CPR* for 2 minutes in a cycle of 30 compressions to 2 effective ventilation breathes.
- After 2 minutes of CPR, check the pulse and assess the rhythm on the monitor.
- If no change in the rhythm, charge and administer the second shock in the same manner as above.

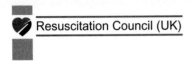

Resuscitation Council (UK)

Adult Advanced Life Support Algorithm

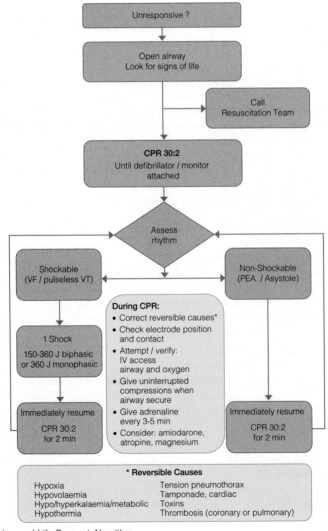

Adult Advanced Life Support Algorithm

- If asystole or pulseless electrical activity, follow the non-shockable rhythm algorithm.
- If organised electrical activity, check for signs of life.
- Continue this cycle, using the time during CPR to assess the underlying cause (as outlined below).
- Before the third shock, administer 1 mg adrenaline (1 in 10 000) IV, and thereafter before every other shock, i.e., before the fifth, seventh, nineth shock etc.
- Before the fourth shock, administer 300 mg amiodarone IV (once only).

Precordial thump

If delivered *within 30 seconds* of a cardiac arrest, a precordial thump is a known, effective method a converting VF or pulseless VT into sinus rhythm. It should however only be used when the arrest is *witnessed and monitored*.

Non-shockable rhythms

- Asystole:
  - Absent QRS waves; P waves may persist
  - Fine VF should be treated as asystole
- Pulseless electrical activity
  - Electrical activity displayed on the trace that is associated with a cardiac output in normal circumstances
  - No palpable pulse in patient.

For non-shockable rhythms:

- *Immediately resume CPR* for 2 minutes in a cycle of 30 compressions to 2 effective ventilation breaths.
- *Immediately* administer 1 mg adrenaline (1 in 10 000) IV, and thereafter every 3–5 minutes
- *Immediately* administer 3 mg atropine IV if in asystole or pulseless electrical activity with rate less than 60/min
- After 2 minutes of CPR, check the pulse and assess the rhythm on the monitor:
  - If no change in the rhythm, continue with two minutes of CPR as above
  - If VF or pulseless VT, follow shockable rhythm algorithm
  - If organised electrical activity, check for signs of life.
- Continue this cycle, using the time during CPR to assess the underlying cause (as outlined below)

During CPR

- Check leads are well sited and that contact is adequate.
- Instruct the anaesthetist to intubate the patient. Subsequently, compressions and ventilation breaths can be asynchronous – compressions at a rate of 100/min, ventilations at a rate of 12/min.
- Ensure IV access is obtained (two large wide bore cannulae into each anterior cubital fossa – take baseline FBC, U&Es and cross match blood).
- Ensure an arterial blood gas is performed.
- If not already present, request that the patient's notes be obtained.
- Request a temperature and blood pressure reading.

Investigate underlying reversible causes of cardiac arrest

- **Hypoxia:** administer oxygen
- **Hypovolaemia:** give any form of fluid resuscitation
- **Hyperkalaemia:** IV calcium gluconate, 50% IV insulin/dextrose
- **Hypokalaemia:** 20–40 ml potassium diluted in 100 ml of NaCl (0.9%)
- **Hypothermia:** warm , e.g., with warmed fluids, blankets
- **Tension pneumothorax:** difficult to anaesthetise, is chest movement and air entry equal?
- **Tamponade:** has the patient been stabbed or are the has there been recent signs of cardiac surgery?
- **Thromboembolic event:** consider thrombolysis
- **Toxic disturbance:** administer antidote if known, call for advice if unknown.

Post resuscitation

Ensure the following checklist is completed following a successful resuscitation:

- A – arterial blood gas (ABG)
- B – baseline bloods, i.e., full blood count (FBC), urea and electrolytes (U&Es), liver function tests (LFTs), cross match
- C – chest X-ray
- D – discharging the patient, i.e., arrange transfer of the patient, for example, to ward/ITU
- E – electrocardiogram (ECG)
- F – family, i.e., inform any relatives of the current situation
- G – Gratitude, i.e., thank the team with which you have been working.

⊙ The Critically Ill Patient

Examiner's instruction

"You are on wards and have been asked to assess a critically patient, Mrs Samantha Jones. Present your findings from the assessment to your examiner."

Before addressing the patient, gather as much information as possible, including:
* Any significant events leading up to this deterioration in health – e.g., postoperative patient
* Any known past medical history – e.g., known diabetic
* Any known vital observations – pulse rate, blood pressure, respiratory rate, oxygen saturation, temperature, urine output
* If possible, request that someone bring you the patient's notes and drug chart.

Danger
* Wash your hands.
* Is it safe to approach the area – is there any immediate danger to yourself or the patient such as blood or spillages or needles.

Response
* Approach the patient
* Assess level of responsiveness by talking to the patient

The ABCDE approach
Assessment of the critically ill patient involves an ABCDE approach

A – Airway

Causes of airway obstruction can include the tongue, foreign bodies, vomit, blood or swelling due to anaphylaxis or trauma.

- **Look:** for any obvious obstructions
- **Feel:** for breath over the mouth
- **Listen:** for stridor/ wheeze/ snoring/ gargling
- **Treat:**
  - Clear any obstructions visible using suction if necessary
  - Head tilt/chin lift to open the airway
  - Airway adjuncts.

Talking to the patient allows for a good assessment of the patient's airway patency – if they are able to form a coherent reply, they are likely to have a patent airway.

B – Breathing

- **Look:**
  - Cyanosis/ pursed lips/ nasal flaring
  - Use of accessory respiratory muscles
- **Feel:**
  - Tracheal tug/ tracheal deviation
  - Symmetrical chest expansion
  - Percuss over the chest for areas of hyper-resonance/dullness
- **Listen:** symmetry of air entry and any wheeze or crackles
- **Measure:**
  - Respiratory rate
  - Oxygen saturation
  - Arterial blood gas
  - Peak flow if appropriate
- **Treat:**
  - Oxygen (high flow, 10–15 l/min) through a non-rebreath mask and reservoir bag) to ensure saturations are above 85%.
  - Administer salbutamol nebuliser if appropriate
  - Arrange a chest X-ray.

C – Circulation

- **Look:**
  - Pallor
  - Pale/ cold/ clammy patient
  - Assess the JVP for signs of volume overload
  - Ankle oedema and sacral oedema
  - Signs of a DVT

* **Feel:**
  - The temperature of the peripheries
  - The character of the pulse
* **Listen:** heart sounds, any murmurs and added sounds
* **Measure:**
  - Pulse rate
  - Blood pressure
  - Capillary refill
  - Urine output
  - Temperature
  - Arrange an ECG
* **Treat:**
  * Gain IV access using two wide bore cannula via each anterior cubital fossa
  * Take bloods for FBC, U&Es, cross match, group and save
  * Administer a fluid challenge (250 mls of colloid over 20 minutes)
  * Order O negative blood if appropriate
  * Assess the need for antibiotics (if febrile).

D – Disability

Assessing disability involves a rapid overview of the patient's current neurological state.

* **Look:**
  * Patient's general state of consciousness
  * Pupillary response to light
  * Assess where the patient lies on the AVPU scale:
    * A – alert
    * V – responding to voice
    * P – responding to a painful stimuli
    * U – unresponsive
* **Measure:** blood glucose level
* **Treat:**
  * If BM less than 3 mmols, administer 25–50 ml 50% glucose IV
  * Assess the need for analgesia, e.g., IV morphine.

At this point, repeat and review the patient's vital observations to assess whether any treatment implemented has had any beneficial effect.

E – Expose the patient

Expose the patient completely and check for any immediate signs:
* Palpate the abdomen
* Bleeding from any wounds
* Roll the patient to the side if appropriate and inspect the leg

- Contact the relevant medical staff involved in his care and/or specialist from whom you would like a review
- Review the patient's notes and drug chart
- If possible, obtain a history from the patient and/or nursing staff
- Review previous investigations that have been performed.

Documentation

In the patient's notes, document:

- The event
- The patient's vital observations
- Findings on examination
- Any actions undertaken

Critical care outreach teams

Most hospitals have a trained outreach team that can be contacted when a team is dealing with critically ill patients. They provide support and assistance in helping medical staff manage such patients. Each hospital has a set of criteria that advise when it may be appropriate to call on these teams.

Administrating Oxygen Therapy

Examiner's instruction

"Mr. Elliott Top has been admitted in respiratory distress. His saturations are 85% in air. Deliver the correct amount of oxygen via the appropriate method. Explain how you would monitor Mr. Top and prescribe the oxygen you are delivering."

ACE TIPS

* Ensure you give oxygen through the correct device and that you fit it properly to the patient.

* Be aware of how to prescribe oxygen.

Indications of oxygen therapy

Oxygen therapy aims to deliver oxygen to a patient at a higher concentration than that found in room air (>21%). The purpose of oxygen therapy is to raise a patient's oxygen saturation to *above 90%*.

Indications for adult oxygen therapy are as follows:

* SpO_2 < 92% on room air
* During acute attacks, e.g., myocardial infarction, haemorrhage, acute asthma
* As prophylaxis of hypoxaemia, e.g., post anaesthesia
* During or recovery from exertion/exercise
* Long term home oxygen therapy for specific chronic conditions

Prescribing oxygen

Oxygen is considered to be a drug and, therefore, it must be prescribed as with any other form of therapy administered to a patient. The following should be documented in both the patient notes and drug chart:

* The device used for oxygen delivery (see below)
* The SpO_2 level that is to be maintained in the patient, e.g., "SpO_2 > 90%"
* The parameters of flow rate or percentage oxygen that nursing staff may fluctuate between in order to maintain optimum saturation
* Frequency of observations.

Oxygen delivery systems

Oxygen is supplied from a source by the patient's bedside and connected via oxygen tubing to one of a variety of available masks, worn by the patient. The bedside source may be manipulated to alter the flow (litres/minute) of oxygen. An appropriate mask should be prescribed as this can determine the percentage oxygen attained by each breath.

- Bag valve mask device – ventilates with ambient air only, thus at a concentration of 21%. Commonly used to manually ventilate apnoeic patients or those with irregular respiration
- Variable percentage mask – with this, the final concentration of oxygen inspired cannot be accurately determined and may vary between approximately 25 and 50%. Determining factors include the applied oxygen flow rate and the depth/rate of the patients respiration
  - E.g., nasal cannula – provides low flow oxygen (2–4 l/min) at a concentration of 28–44%. It is often used in elderly patients, patients requiring minimal oxygen therapy or those patients who cannot tolerate wearing an oxygen mask
- Standard oxygen mask – approximately 45% oxygen can be administered at 5–6 l/min
  - A reservoir bag may be applied to the standard oxygen mask in order to increase the concentration of oxygen available to the patient (up to approximately 80% at 10–15 l/min). It is generally used in critically ill patients
- Fixed percentage masks – oxygen first passes through a device attached to the mask, before reaching the patient. When the flow is set to the rate stated upon the mask, the device accurately controls the percentage of oxygen available to the patient. This is useful in situations where the control of oxygen inspired is crucial, such as during the management of chronic obstructive airway disease (where masks administering only 24–28% oxygen are generally used to prevent CO_2 retention)
  - E.g., venturi mask – delivers fixed oxygen concentrations of 24–60% depending on the mask selected.

Monitoring
Whilst patients are undergoing oxygen therapy, 4-hourly observations including respiratory rate and SpO_2 should be undertaken.

Precautions
- Patients with chronic obstructive lung disease must be carefully monitored via arterial blood gas analysis – this is in order to minimise the risk of CO_2 retention whilst ensuring reversal of hypoxaemia.
- Prolonged use of oxygen therapy (>12 hours) without added humidification can adversely affect cilia and the production of mucous within the respiratory tract.
- Patients should be made aware of the dangers of smoking near oxygen delivering equipment due to the high risk of combustion.
- Healthcare staff should be informed of how to manage oxygen therapy during circumstances in which it can be potentially dangerous, such as defibrillation.

If a subsequent rise in $PaCO_2$ to dangerous levels (greater or equal to 9 kPa) ensues as a direct result of oxygen therapy, interventions such as ventilatory support or respiratory stimulants are indicated.

⚙ Basic Airway Management

Examiner's instructions

"A patient is admitted to the Accident & Emergency Department with a reduced level of consciousness leading the staff to be concerned about his airway. Assess the situation and take the appropriate action."

- **D** – check for danger, wash hands and put on any protective equipment (gloves, apron)
- **R** – assess the patients response: the patient moans on a verbal cue
- **A** – look in airway for signs of airway obstruction.

The examiner states: *"There is blood and vomit in the patient's mouth."*
- Suggest recovery position (if not concerned about C-spine injury and choose the Yankaeur sucker (oral suction catheter) to clear upper airway. When using Yankaeur demonstrate clearing from side to side, always being able to visualise end of suction tube.

The examiner states: *"The airway is now clear of blood and vomit."*
- Listen for noises – stridor, gurgling, wheeze, snoring, choking.

The examiner states: *"You hear a snoring noise and look in the mouth to see a carrot obstructing the airway.*
- Select the Magill forceps to remove the obstruction

The examiner states: *"O₂ saturations are recorded to show 89%."*
- Select and apply oxygen via Hudson mask with oxygen reservoir bag, mentioning that this will deliver high concentration (80%+) oxygen.

The examiner states: *"The patient has begun to make snoring noises again and has dropped his conscious level (no response from patient), and sats have dropped back down to 90%."*
- Recognise need for airway, selecting oropharyngeal airway as patient is unconscious. The airway is sized by measuring from the corner mouth to tragus of ear; select correct size, insert in upside-down position and rotate into place.

The examiner asks: *"If no equipment was available, what basic airway manoeuvre would be indicated?"*
- Head tilt/chin lift – demonstrate.

The examiner asks: *"What manoeuvre would be indicated if the patient was at risk of a C-spine injury?"*

• Jaw thrust – demonstrate.

The examiner asks: *"Which adjunct could you alternatively select if the patient had a gag reflex?"*

• Select and name nasopharyngeal airway – measure by estimating size of nostril to diameter of adjunct.

The examiner states: *"The patient has now stopped breathing. What piece of equipment would you use?"*

• Select and name bag valve mask to mechanically ventilate patient; remember to ask for assistance to use BVM. Ensure the mask is secure, and the helper must squeeze bag, . delivering approximately 500 ml, 14 breaths per minute.

ACE TIP

Remember to call for help at any stage (such as medical emergency team)

Completing a Hospital Discharge Form

Patient details

In most hospital units you will be provided with pre-printed patient "addressograph" labels. However, in an examination setting you may be asked to complete the patient's details by hand. Make sure to complete the patient's:

- Full name and date of birth
- Hospital number and/or NHS number
- Address

Admission details

The following admission details are important to document:

- Date of admission
- Route of admission (e.g., via accident and emergency; direct admission, via outpatients, transfer from another hospital etc.)
- Named consultant
- Hospital and ward to which the patient was admitted.

Clinical condition(s)

Often there maybe more than one condition for which a patient was admitted to hospital. Therefore, in order of clinical importance, document all conditions that contributed to the patients' admission. When recording a clinical diagnosis try to use correct medical terminology (e.g., use "inferior myocardial infraction" rather than "heart attack"). Most hospitals use a clinical coding system that will help you to code accurately and also assign a correct code identity. This is important in terms of audit and monitoring of disease incidence and prevalence.

Operations and/or procedures

Be sure to document any operations, procedures and/or important investigations that the patient had during their hospital admission. Also, record the date of when these activities were carried out, as this may be different from the date of admission. Often students overlook certain investigations as "not being important" (e.g., exercise stress test, echocardiography, CT/ MRI), however, such information is important to record, particularly for the GP quality outcomes framework.

Drugs on discharge

This is one of the most important sections of the discharge form. It is vital that you take time to accurately record all relevant details about a patient's medication on discharge. Any mistakes in such recording may result in a medication error that could potentially harm the patient.

For each drug that the patient is to be discharged on, make sure to document:

- Full name of drug
- Dose and correct units
- Route of administration (e.g., oral, inhaled, transdermal, per rectum, subcutaneous)
- Frequency of administration (e.g., once daily, twice daily, once weekly)
- Whether medication is to be used on demand (e.g., twice daily when required, two puffs with onset of chest pain)

- Duration of course (e.g., one week, one month, long term, until review)
- Whether a supply of the drug has been given to the patient, and if so the amount that was supplied.

It is also good practice to highlight to the patient's GP, which drugs were either:

- Newly started during their admission
- Changed (e.g., dose either increased or decreased)
- Unchanged
- Discontinued.

ACE TIPS

- Make sure that your handwriting is clear and legible.

- Never use a pencil. Black pen should be used ideally.

- Avoid medical abbreviations.

- Write drug names in capital letters.

- Where appropriate record generic names of drugs.

- If patients have been prescribed hypnotics *only* during their admission, make sure to discontinue them after discharge.

Medical summary

Most discharge forms allow for a short clinical summary about the patient's admission. It is good practice to record:

- The main reasons for the patient's admission
- How the patient was managed and any decisions that where made
- Any significant events that occurred during their admission
- Are there any outstanding investigations and/or procedures to be performed after the patient has been discharged?
- Any action points that one would like the GP to do once the patient has been discharged, for example:
  - Whether the patient should make an appointment with their GP
  - Perform any blood tests
  - Address any outstanding clinical issues after discharge (e.g., a patient was found to be hypertensive during their admission and you would like their GP to follow this up)
  - Notification of any other allied healthcare professionals (such as district nurse, social worker, practice nurse).

Review arrangements

If the patient is to be reviewed at hospital again, make sure to record:

- Duration until next review
- Place of review (e.g., outpatient department, day ward, readmission date for a procedure).

Discharge details

Ensure that you record:

• Date of discharge

• Where the patient was discharged to (e.g., own home, nursing home, other ward, other hospital).

Doctor's details

Finally you should record your own details on the discharge form. It is good practice to record the following information:

• Printed name

• Your grade (e.g., FY1, FY2)

• Your contact number or bleep number

• Date and signature.

Example OSCE station

Examiner's instruction

"Please read the following clinical summary and complete the patient's hospital discharge form."

ACE TIPS

• Typically in such stations you will be provided with a clinical summary of a patient's hospital admission, a copy of their drug chart and a blank discharge form

• Ensure you read the question properly and fill in all the necessary information correctly.

Clinical summary

Patient details:

Mr John Smith, DOB 16/12/1961
Address: 1 The Street, Anytown.
Hospital number: 07/01234
You are a FY1 doctor (bleep number 007) who works on ward 10, St Elsewhere Hospital.
Your consultant is Mr F Flinstone.

Mr John Smith was admitted to your ward on 10 October 2007, via the Accident and Emergency department. He presented with severe abdominal pain, haematemsis and maelena. He had an oesophago-gastro-duodenoscopy (OGD) performed on the same day, which revealed severe gastritis. He was commenced on a proton pump inhibitor (omeprazole 20 mg, once daily) and settled with analgesia. On admission his haemoglobin count was 7.5 g/dl and he was transfused 4 units of blood in the Accident and Emergency department.

He has a history of knee osteoarthritis and had been taking long term NSAIDs – which presumably caused his gastritis. His NSAIDs were discontinued and he was commenced on paracetamol (500–1000 mg) every 4–6 hours on a when-required basis. He is to stay on omperazole until his next hospital review. Pharmacy supplied him with (28) omperazole 20 mg tablets and (60) 500 mg paracetamol tablets.

He is to be discharged home today, 14 October 2007, and is due for review in 6 weeks in the endoscopy unit, for a repeat OGD. You would like the GP to repeat his FBC in 2 weeks to ensure that his blood count hasn't dropped any further. His haemoglobin was 13.6 g/dl on discharge.

Completed discharge form

Figure 69.1 shows the completed form.

Patient details	Hospital / ward details
Mr John Smith DOB 16/12/1961	Ward 10, St Elsewhere
Address: 1 The Street, Anytown	**Consultant**
Hospital number: 07/01234	Mr F Flinstone

Admission details	
Date of admission: 10/10/07	Date of discharge: 14/10/07
Admitted from: Accident and emergency	Discharged to: Home

Diagnosis:

1) Upper gastrointestinal haemorrhage

2) Non steroidal anti-inflammatory drug induced gastritis

3) Osteoarthritis of knee

Operation/ Procedures

1) Oesophagogastroendoscopy (10/10/07)

2) Blood transfusion (10/10/07)

DRUGS ON DISCHARGE

DRUG	DOSE	ROUTE	FREQUENCY	DURATION OF COURSE	NUMBER OF TABLETS SUPPLIED
OMEPRAZOLE (New)	20mg	ORAL	ONCE DAILY	UNTIL REPEAT OGD IN 6 WEEKS	28
PARACETMOL (New)	500mg - 1g	ORAL	EVERY 4-6 HOURS WHEN REQUIRED	INDEFINITELY	60

SUMMARY

45year old patient admitted with upper GI bleed. Stabilized in accident and emergency; Initial Hb 7.5 g/dl - received 4 units of blood. OGD revealed gastritis. Known history OA of knees and on long term NSAID. Commenced on omperazole and fit for discharge. Hb on discharge 13.6 g/dl. To continue on omperazole until repeat OGD in 6 weeks. Please could you 1) STOP NSAIDS. 2) check FBC in 2 weeks time to ensure blood count hasn't dropped any further.

REVIEW ARRANGEMENTS	To attend endoscopy unit as day patient in 6 weeks time
DOCTOR DETAILS	Dr B Rubble FY1 doctor Bleep 007
SIGNATURE *Dr B Rubble*	**DATE** 14/10/07

Hospital discharge form

Completing a Warfarin Hospital Discharge Form

Patient details

In most hospital units you will be provided with preprinted patient "addressograph" labels. However, in an examination setting you may be asked to complete the patient's details by hand. Make sure to complete the patient's:

- Full name and date of birth
- Hospital number and/or NHS number
- Address.

Admission details

The following admission details are important to document:

- Date of admission
- Named consultant
- Hospital ward or clinic to which the patient was admitted.

Clinical summary

It is good practice to summarize the patient's clinical history:

- Exact clinical diagnosis (e.g., distal DVT, proximal DVT, pulmonary embolus, recurrent DVT, recurrent pulmonary embolus, atrial fibrillation, mitral or aortic valve disease, cardiomyopathy, tissue heart replacement valve, mechanical prosthetic valve)
- How they presented clinically
- How they where investigated (for example d-dimer blood test, duplex ultrasound scan, venogram).

Anticoagulation history

Spend time to accurately and legibly document the patient's prescribed anticoagulation history. This should include:

- If the patient was prescribed low molecular weight heparin:
  - Date commenced
  - Duration
  - Date discontinued
- All information in relation to warfarin that has been prescribed including:
  - Date commenced
  - Each daily dose prescribed, together with date.

Recommended target INR and INR range

These values will depend on the individual clinical case and local guidelines. It is important to convey:

- The target INR value for that patient (e.g., proximal DVT, target INR ~2.5; mechanical prosthetic heart valve, target INR ~3.0)
- Acceptable INR range (e.g., atrial fibrillation ~2.0–3.0).

Expected duration of warfarin treatment

This will depend on the individual clinical case and local hospital guidelines for anticoagulation (e.g., pulmonary embolus, ~6 months; cardiomyopathy, life long).

Discharge details

Ensure that you record:

- Date of discharge
- Daily dose of warfarin that the patient should take until their next INR check
- When the patient is due to have their next INR checked
- Who is to perform the next INR check (e.g., anticoagulation clinic, GP treatment room nurse, district nurse).

Review arrangements

If the patient is to be reviewed at hospital again, make sure to record:

- Duration until next review
- Place of review (e.g., outpatient department, anticoagulation clinic).

Patient counselling

It is good practice to document that a patient has been:

- Counselled about warfarin therapy
- Issued with a personal warfarin monitoring book.

Doctor's details

Finally, you should record your own details on the discharge form. It is good practice to record the following information:

- Printed name
- Your grade (e.g., FY1, FY2)
- Your contact number or bleep number
- Date and signature.

ACE TIPS

- Make sure that your handwriting is clear and legible.

- Never use a pencil. A black pen is advised.

- Avoid abbreviations.

- Make sure any decimal points are quite clearly indicated (e.g., do not confuse 1.0 mg with 10 mg).

- Consider who will perform the patient's next INR check and when it will be – remember getting an INR checked on a Sunday in the community may not be straight forward.

- For immobile patients who are discharged into the community, it is good practice to inform the GP and the district nursing team about the patients discharge arrangements.

Example OSCE station

Examiner's instruction

"Please read the following clinical summary and complete the patient's warfarin hospital discharge."

Clinical summary

Patient details:

Mrs Mary Smith, DOB 1/10/1941
Address: 1 The Close, Anycity
Hospital number: 07/43210
Consultant: Dr B Stoker, Accident and Emergency department.

You are a FY2 doctor (page number 001) who works in the Accident and Emergency department of St Elsewhere's Hospital. Mrs Mary Smith was admitted to the department with a painful swollen, tender right calf on the 23/8/07. Clinically you suspected a DVT. The patient's d-dimer test came back elevated at 9.98 µg/ml. A duplex ultrasound scan confirmed a right distal DVT. She was commenced on low molecular heparin on 23/08/07 and prescribed warfarin as shown in the table below.

DATE	23/8/07	24/8/07	25/08/07	26/8/07	27/8/07	28/8/07	29/8/07	30/08/07
DOSE	10 mg	10 mg	5 mg	5 mg	5 mg	5 mg	5 mg	–
INR	1.01	–	2.01	2.29	–	2.43	–	Due

The patient had her low molecular weight heparin discontinued on 25/8/07. The patient's target INR is 2.5 with a range of 2.0–3.0. The consultant intends to stop the warfarin after 3 months. The patient is to be discharged from the Accident and Emergency department's and care is to be transferred to the general practitioner on 28/08/07. You have counselled the patient about warfarin and have given them their warfarin monitoring book. They are due to have their next INR performed on the 30/08/07 at their GP practice.

Completed warfarin discharge form

Figure 70.1 shows the completed form.

Patient details:	Hospital / ward details:
Mrs Mary Smith 1/10/1941	Accident and Emergency Department, St Elsewhere
Address: 1 The Close, Anycity	**Consultant:**
Hospital number: 07/43210	Dr B Stoker
Admission details	
Date of admission: 23/8/07	Date of discharge: 28/8/07
Admitted from: Accident and Emergency to DVT clinic	Discharged to: Home and Care of General Practitioner

Clinical summary and diagnosis:

Patient admitted with swollen, tender right calf. D-dimer elevated at 9.98 µg/ml. Duplex ultrasound confirmed presence of right distal DVT. Commenced on enoxaparin on 23/8/07 and stopped on 25/08/07.

Warfarin dosing as follows:

DATE	23/8/07	24/8/07	25/08/07	26/8/07	27/8/07	28/8/07	29/8/07	30/08/07
DOSE	10 mg	10 mg	5.0 mg	5.0 mg	5.0 mg	5.0 mg	5.0 mg	-
INR	1.01	-	2.01	2.29	-	2.43	-	*Due*

Indication	Distal deep venous thrombosis
Target INR	2.5
INR range	2.0 – 3.0
Duration of warfarin therapy	3 months
Next INR due	30/08/07
Warfarin counselling received?	Yes
Warfarin monitoring book issued?	Yes
Review arrangements	GP to follow up. No routine follow-up in Accident and Emergency department/ DVT clinic. Patient knows to make appointment with GP and practice nurse
Doctor details	Dr H Simpson, FY2 doctor, Bleep 001.
Signature Dr H Simpson	**Date** 28/08/07

Hospital warfarin discharge form

Verification of Death and Death Certificate

Confirming life extinct and certifying the medical cause of death may appear as an OSCE station in medical finals. This is a commonly performed act by foundation year doctors and, therefore, ripe to appear in final examinations. Like any other procedure you should have a systematic approach for how to verify death and complete, if appropriate, a medical certificate of the cause of death. There are many guidelines of how to diagnose death. In all circumstances you must perform a thorough physical examination to ascertain whether or not death has taken place and any particular information related to that patient's death. It is worth noting that there are certain circumstances (e.g., hypothermia; after ingestion of alcohol or drugs; hypoglycaemia or after being in a coma) where a detailed examination is required to fully ensure whether death has actually occurred.

In most cases, a doctor can certify the medical cause of death. This is a statutory form and therefore you should take time to complete it fully and accurately. Once this form is forwarded to the Registrar of Births, Deaths and Marriages then death can be registered. Typically in such OSCE stations you will be provided with a short clinical summary of the case, a mannequin to demonstrate how you would confirm death and a blank death certificate.

Verification of death

Inspect

- Take time to inspect the external appearance of the deceased. Observe for any external clinical signs or signs of trauma. It is also worth noting the external environment immediate to the deceased.

- Inspect the deceased's pupils for their size, symmetry and shape. Now examine with a bright torch for any pupillary reflexes (i.e., in a deceased patient you would expect fixed dilated pupils).

- You may consider examining for other reflexes including the corneal, gag and/or vestibulo-ocular reflexes.

Palpate

- Now palpate for the carotid pulse for at least 1 minute.

Auscultate

- For at least 1 minute, listen over the praecordium for any heart sounds.
- Auscultate over the chest for at least 1 minute for any breath sounds.

Documentation

- Record your findings accurately, including the date and time that life was pronounced extinct.

Certification of death

Consider whether the Coroner needs to notified of the death

- Consider this prior to completing the death certificate. Circumstances in which to notify the Coroner differ slightly from region to region. You should familiarise yourself with these circumstances.

Patient details

You will need to complete the following patient details on the death certificate:

- Full name of the deceased
- Usual residence of the deceased
- Place of death
- Date of death
- Health service number of the deceased (if known).

Cause of death

It is vital that you accurately record the exact cause of death. You should avoid using any abbreviations, nonmedical terminology or symptoms (e.g., shortness of breath, chest pain). You will need to document the following:

- The disease or condition that directly led to the patients death
- Any antecedent causes
- Any other significant conditions contributing to the death, but not related to the disease or condition causing it.

Details of the relevant medical practitioner(s)

The following details also need to be completed:

- Date when last seen alive and treated by the practitioner for the fatal illness
- Whether seen after death by the practitioner or by another medial practitioner
- Certifying doctors full name and signature
- Certifying doctors place of work
- Certifying doctors qualifications as registered by the GMC
- Date of certificate completed.

ACE TIPS

- Make sure to inform relevant family members of the deceased's death.

- It is good practice to telephone the patient's GP at the earliest opportunity to confirm the death of a patient from their list.

- Make sure you cancel any prearranged hospital appointments that the deceased may of had.